SLEEP
MATTERS

the yawn of a new day!

JoAnn Cutler Friedrich, P.A.

Bright Books
4718 Meridian Avenue, Suite 212
San Jose, California 95118
(408) 266-1400

Book Design by Katharine Ford
Sage Media

Cover Graphics by Daniel L. Burney
Ideas In Print

Dedication

With love to my daughter, Jill
and my husband, Michael.
May all your hopes and dreams come true.

Contents

Order Form

1 *Sleep Debt*

A National Deficit and Growing

Z Z Z Z Z Z Z Z Z Z Z Z Z Z Z Z Z Z Z Z Z Z Z Z Z

If you're like most people, you care about the environment and the national debt. You're aware of the many problems facing this country today, but you're just too tired and stressed to do anything about them. The average person works far too many hours. And the wear and tear this lifestyle has caused are beginning to show not only on the individual, but on society as a whole.

It shouldn't surprise you to learn that millions of people aren't getting enough sleep. Chances are, you're probably one of them. In which case, you're already experiencing the effects of what many experts have come to view as a national epidemic of sleep loss.

Stanford University sleep researcher, William Dement (who is credited with many of the earliest studies of dream states and their role in promoting health and well-being), has emerged as a passionate advocate of the benefits of sleep. "Most Americans don't know what it feels like to be fully alert," (he has said.) "So many of us fail to get the proper amount of sleep that I would say we have a new kind of national debt to worry about, a national sleep debt, one that is no less dangerous to our economy, our security and our well-being than the monetary one."

Cover stories in *Time* and other leading publications and feature articles in men's, women's, parent's, business and health magazines are focusing the nation's attention on this serious problem. Leading authorities on sleep, such as Dement, are blatantly telling us that most people aren't sleeping enough, and even more of us aren't getting the quality of sleep we need. Not surprisingly, the blame for this nation-wide burnout is placed on inadequate night-time sleep.

The problem of sleep loss is now perceived to be so acute that the U.S. Congress recently commissioned a study on the nation's sleep habits. The results were sobering. "Sleep deprivation is pervasive throughout our society," says a 1993 report of the National Commission on Sleep Disorders Research. According to the federal study, an estimated 50 million American adults (just adults, mind you) frequently or chronically complain about sleep. Of these, half are plagued by insomnia and the rest suffer from daytime sleepiness. As many as 100 million Americans may suffer from daytime drowsiness. By his count, it's safe to assume that some 60 million women and 40 million men in the United States today suffer from sleep problems.

From this study, you can see just how big the problem is, but you're probably wondering how sleep loss affects you. Interestingly, sleep deprivation is one of the most critical factors in mental well-being. I'd say that 100 million tired people translates into an epidemic of unhappiness in America, at a staggering cost in terms of our creativity and productivity.

Today, the United States ranks second only to Japan among industrialized nations afflicted by insufficient sleep. And while in Japan the problem is so acute that there's even a Japanese word, *karoshi* (death from overwork), exhaustion is increasingly recognized as a health problem with severe repercussions for our own society as well.

The national sleep debt is big business, too. All over the country, sleep disorder clinics are springing up like weeds, more than 200 to date, and the numbers are growing (see Appendix A). Ten million plus Americans see a doctor for sleep problems every year, and half of those leave the doctor's office with a prescription for an expensive sleep medication. Ironically, most of this medicine further compounds the problem. We are spending enormous sums of money each year on prescription and over-the-counter medications which, their manufacturers assure us, will either put us to sleep or rouse us from the drowsy effects of getting too little sleep.

The hidden costs of the national sleep debt are also enormous. Estimates of poor sleep habits and its expense to industry (and in the work place in general) vary widely. But the collective impact on our society is clearly astronomical in financial terms.

Our national sleep epidemic has a destructive toll on our safety as well. More and more studies show that daytime drowsiness is a leading cause of traffic fatalities and industrial mishaps.

According to the Department of Transportation, as many as 400,000 traffic accidents each year may be related to sleepiness. Even more staggering, between 8,000 and 10,000 of these are fatalities.

Viewed historically, healthful sleep has been the casualty of a radical shift in the way we lead our lives. Prior to the invention of the lightbulb, some would say before the invention of fire, man awoke and slept according to the natural progression from day to night and back again. For example, accounts from Elizabethan times of major festivities mention roistering crowds who stayed up until ten o'clock as an indication of the intense excitement generated by these celebrations.

Even 100 years ago before the popularization of the electric lightbulb by Thomas Edison (a notoriously light sleeper who boasted of needing only a few hours sleep a night, while he slipped frequent naps into his daily schedule), people were still sleeping on average of about nine and a half hours. Nowadays, most of us are lucky if we get anywhere from five to seven hours of uninterrupted sleep per night. Researchers estimate, and it's a conservative estimate in my opinion, that the majority of Americans get between 60 to 90 minutes less sleep each night than they should.

Sleep deprivation is something most of us think of in terms of brainwashing and mind control by covert military operations and guerilla factions. That's exactly what's happening to many of us each and every day on a smaller scale. Chronically sleep deprived, we are routinely bombarded with images of what we should look like and how we should live. Confused and disoriented by this barrage of unrealistic information, we feel cheated and disappointed when the facts of our lives fall short of our fantasies.

Not surprisingly, there is a rapidly mounting body of evidence which shows that sleep deprivation has become one of the most pervasive mental health problems facing the nation today. Extreme sleep loss may result in hallucinations, brief durations of sleep during the waking state known as "microsleep", and such behavioral syndromes as acute suspicion and fear. Moderate sleep deprivation mimics the same paranoidal tendencies in more subtle, unrecognized ways.

Other observers have noted another insidious consequence of the sleep debt, namely the underlying irritation that seems to consume more and more people every day. Anyone who has commuted during a big city morning rush hour can understand what I'm talking about. More frightening is the pathological behavior, either abusive, criminal or downright murderous, which I believe is often triggered by long-term disturbed patterns of sleep. It is my belief that our society has severely underplayed the social costs of troubled sleep, and we are doing so at our own peril.

Becoming aware of the scope of this problem first requires some personal self-examination. At least one expert has suggested that if you have to get up by six a.m., you're probably already sleep deprived. The same goes if you find you get up much later on weekend mornings than during the week, or even if you feel more burned out on Friday than you do after the weekend.

Maybe you still don't believe you're sleep deprived. Just answer the following question. Do you have an alarm clock to wake you up? If you have to set the alarm at night, you're sleep deprived. It's that simple. I might add that the lucrative market for snooze buttons on bedside clocks, a modern form of psychological torture if you want my opinion, is just another symptom of our national sleep debt.

Sleep deprivation is also cumulative. This means your personal sleep debt builds up over time because sleep loss accumulates night after night. Sleep loss takes its toll before most of us notice the effects because we have instinctively learned how to compensate for sleepiness in our daily functioning.

For most people, a good night's sleep is more and more viewed as a kind of reward, something you do for yourself after you've spent a busy work week without getting enough sleep. Unfortunately, by the time you get enough sleep, the damage has already been done.

The fact is you can never really "catch up on your sleep." Although a few well-publicized studies have suggested that performance isn't impaired by mild sleep deprivation, newer research challenges this notion. Even one night of inadequate sleep can produce obvious physiological and cognitive imbalances. The next day, you can still expect to respond for short periods of time to the immediate demands of a situation, but your mental concentration, flexibility, and creativity (the ability to deal spontaneously and imaginatively to problems), has already suffered. Losing sleep for a single night has been proven to diminish your ability to think creatively during the day, and the same lack of sleep is known to affect your ability to execute more routine tasks by later in that afternoon.

After a second night of insufficient sleep, you can expect even rote functioning to be uniformly affected. By the end of an average working week, your performance and functioning can be seriously impaired. Prolonged sleep loss can also injure your body's innate and well-documented ability to fight off illness and heal mental and physical damage.

Contrary to what you may have been led to believe, there's no way to balance your sleep debt other than by getting more sleep. Diet, exercise, various forms of rest (meditation, biofeedback), and optimum physical fitness can help you achieve better sleep, but cannot replace it. And many of the factors people blame for feeling tired, heavy meals, repetitive tasks, stuffy surroundings, do not have the same effect on people who get optimal sleep.

What is optimal sleep? Pure and simple, it's the sleep you need to be fully alert in the daytime. And it's not just the amount of sleep that's important. The quality of sleep, which is insufficiently understood by most of us, is also vital.

While the concept of optimal sleep might seem easy enough to grasp, this ideal is still something most of us seem to feel we can do without to some degree or another. Given all the demands on our time and energy from the pressures of modern society, sleep just isn't much of a priority for most people. Experts euphemistically refer to this phenomenon as "voluntary sleep reduction", as if we felt we had a choice in the matter. Shorting ourselves on sleep has been blamed on everything from shift work, with the changing sleep and wake schedules entailed, to frequent flying through time zones among business travellers, as well as the changing patterns of sleep as we age.

Coupled with all this is an obvious prejudice in modern society against sleep, what I call "sleep macho". While in so-called "siesta cultures" the afternoon nap is a respected part of daily life, we Americans seem to pride ourselves on how little sleep we get. Just as we frown on other societies where the therapeutic benefits of sufficient sleep are ingrained in popular consciousness. In our own culture, we use *sleep macho* to exert pressure on others who would prefer to get enough sleep. Sometimes people who sleep more than the norm are viewed as inferior and sickly. We like to think of "heavy" sleepers as basically lazy, unmotivated, or even as clinically depressed.

Alongside all this, as I have said, is a widespread lack of appreciation for the benefits of quality sleep. Too often, what little sleep we do get is hampered by the stress and tensions of our waking lives, poor eating habits, stimulants and depressants. And even when we finally do get to bed, there are many other conditions that can mitigate against the healing properties of sleep.

But in spite of all the hand-wringing about our national sleep debt, very little is being done to correct the problem. I believe sleep deprivation is the number one problem facing Americans today. It is affecting every aspect of our lives from children who have learning difficulties to teens who are using drugs and alcohol. It causes premenstrual syndrome in women and physical abusiveness in men. It is making us a nation of moody, irritable and often confused people. It is sapping our creativity, as well as increasing criminal behavior. And, it is devastating to our economy and industry. We all have too much to do and few of us are getting the rest we need in order to get it all done.

One thing you can say about the sleep debt: it's not going to go away overnight. In the meantime, you owe it to yourself, your family, your friends and fellow workers, to do all you can to insure you get the sleep you need. Some of the techniques you can use may surprise you and some are just good common sense. But, by the time you've finished this book, you will be better equipped to make nature's gift of sleep work for you in achieving greater health, success, and happiness—sleep matters!

To find out if you or a family member need more sleep, take the sleep test on the following pages.

Sleep Matters Test

This self-test is to help you determine how severe your sleep deprivation is. Please indicate whether your symptoms are: (1) mild, (2) moderate, (3) severe.

Absence from work/school	1	2	3
Abuse—verbal or physical	1	2	3
Accident-prone	1	2	3
Aggression	1	2	3
Alcohol—decreased tolerance	1	2	3
Alcohol—increased consumption	1	2	3
Anger	1	2	3
Anxiety	1	2	3
Apathy	1	2	3
Appetite increase	1	2	3
Assault	1	2	3
Avoidance of social activities	1	2	3
Backache	1	2	3
Breathlessness or suffocation	1	2	3
Confusion	1	2	3
Cravings for salt	1	2	3
Cravings for sweet	1	2	3
Crying	1	2	3
Depression	1	2	3
Disorientation	1	2	3
Dizziness	1	2	3

Drug abuse	1	2	3
Excitability	1	2	3
Fatigue or lethargy	1	2	3
Feelings of suffocation	1	2	3
Guilt feelings	1	2	3
Headaches—migraine	1	2	3
Headaches—tension	1	2	3
Heart pounding or irregularity	1	2	3
Increased nervous energy	1	2	3
Increased need to sleep	1	2	3
Increased sensitivity to light	1	2	3
Increased sensitivity to sound	1	2	3
Indecision	1	2	3
Insomnia	1	2	3
Intentional self-injury	1	2	3
Irritability	1	2	3
Irrationality	1	2	3
Loneliness	1	2	3
Loss of control (or fear of)	1	2	3
Mood swings	1	2	3
Muscle stiffness	1	2	3
Panic attacks	1	2	3
Paranoia or suspicion	1	2	3
Poor judgment	1	2	3
Poor coordination	1	2	3
Poor concentration	1	2	3

Restlessness	1	2	3
Sex drive—increase or decrease	1	2	3
Shakiness	1	2	3
Sleep disturbance	1	2	3
Suicidal thoughts	1	2	3
Tension	1	2	3
Urge to hit or throw	1	2	3
Weight gain	1	2	3
Withdrawal	1	2	3

Total your score and compare with the ratings below. This will help assess the presence/severity of your sleep problems. Remember this is a general guideline and there can be many variables.

If your total score is:

1 - 5   Your symptoms are mild and probably interfere minimally with your lifestyle—even minimal symptoms can be alleviated—sleep matters!

6-40   You probably have moderate symptoms. This is the category into which most people fall. Most people in this category feel they are just a little more moody, tired or sensitive, you can feel better every day—sleep matters!

41+   You have severe sleep problems. Your concentration is decreased when you're not sleeping well—you wonder if there's something seriously wrong with you. Correcting your sleep problems can change your life—sleep matters!

2 *Generation Gaps*

The Age of Exhaustion

Z Z Z Z Z Z Z Z Z Z Z Z Z Z Z Z Z Z Z Z Z Z Z Z Z

While it's fair to say that most of us are sleep deprived to some extent, it's also important to recognize that the amount of sleep we need (at various times in our lives, and consequently, the quantity and quality of the sleep we're getting), depends largely on age. When members of a family are separated by a generation, the gap in their sleep needs becomes dramatic. When differing sleep needs vary as widely as they do between, say, the rest a young mother needs and the rest her newborn baby requires, one of the most significant of human interactions, the bond between mother and child, is often the casualty.

2 Generation Gaps

When I first met Melanie she was 37 years old, and the mother of a healthy, brand-new baby girl. Obviously, Melanie's was a late pregnancy, in fact, she had been trying unsuccessfully for the past 15 years to have a baby, consulting many different physicians and trying a number of different methods of getting pregnant. Melanie and her husband believed that the only thing they needed to make their dreams come true was a baby. Needless to say, when she eventually did become pregnant, and furthermore, when the delivery of her baby daughter turned out to be quite easy, Melanie and her husband were deeply thrilled.

But once Melanie came home with her new baby, it wasn't long before she began to notice that she was feeling increasingly miserable. The experts like to refer to Melanie's symptoms as postpartum depression, the "baby blues". Ironically, those who study the subject are often at a loss to explain the causes for it. Although, in my opinion, the reason for this all-too-common malady is obvious.

No one was more confused about this unhappy state of affairs than Melanie, herself. She told me, "I just don't understand it. For years, it seems like all I've dreamed about is having a baby. And, now that I have my little girl, I just feel so hopeless and downhearted. I know I still love her, but I just can't seem to help the way I feel."

These feelings persisted and, as time went by, Melanie began getting even more depressed. Then something unexpected happened. Melanie realized that she was beginning to feel something close to actual hatred for her infant daughter. She talked to her women friends who had children and they were as mystified as she was. Normal postpartum depression was one thing. But, the violent emotions sweeping over Melanie were something else altogether.

By the time another month had elapsed, Melanie became convinced she was capable of physically harming her child. She grew so concerned about her murderous intentions towards her baby, she decided to seek professional help. This is when I met her.

I first asked Melanie about the specifics of her sleep situation. As it turned out, her daughter had suffered from colic for weeks at a time. This is hardly an unusual occurrence for newborns. But one that can have devastating repercussions for new mothers, since a baby with colic is often awake and crying constantly. In Melanie's case, the problem was complicated by her husband's promotion. He was working 70 or more hours each week, thus, she felt the baby was solely her responsibility. Furthermore, she felt hiring someone to help out with her daughter just wasn't right, even though money wasn't an issue.

We quickly established that, prior to the birth of her baby, Melanie was consistently getting a good nine hours of sleep each night, while exercising and eating correctly. Physically, she'd been in great shape when she came to term, which probably had a lot to do with her easy delivery. But now she was getting no more than 45 minutes of sleep at a time. Often, she was lucky if she got that much. After many weeks of interrupted rest, her total sleep time was down to approximately two or three hours a night.

Clearly, Melanie needed help. And fast. We decided to try a different approach. I immediately placed her on the program I designed to enhance brain chemical levels (unfor-

tunately the amino acid used in this program was contaminated by the raw materials manufacturer in 1989 and the FDA has not allowed it back on the market—see Appendix B). Next, she consulted a sympathetic pediatrician about ways of moderating her daughter's colic. She then brought in a part-time nurse to take care of the baby at night. And between us, we devised a creative sleep schedule that took into account the nurse's presence while still allowing Melanie to breast feed her baby.

Melanie's improvement was as rapid as it was dramatic. After a very short period of time, she was inwardly happier and outwardly more cheerful. She was soon peacefully absorbed in her infant daughter's rapid changes. Within a few months, Melanie's little girl was sleeping longer. The nurse was needed less and less, and we both felt that any danger had passed. When I last saw her, Melanie was decidedly upbeat about her situation. "You know," she told me, "I think this is the first time I've felt like a real Mom."

So far, this discussion of sleep needs has focused on the problems of adults. But newborns, as well, are subjected to significant stress that may adversely affect their ability to sleep. If conditions are conducive, newborns will sleep an average of 16 to 18 hours a day, usually in short intervals of two to four hours in length.

Researchers on the subject tell us that once a pattern of sleeplessness is established, the habit is very hard to break. This seems to be particularly true for children. By age one, young children probably need no more than 13 to 14 hours of sleep per day, but that much sleep, even with naps, may be hard to come by when an infant is surrounded by the frenetic comings and goings of the typical modern household.

Not surprisingly, some of the most disturbing childhood behaviors occur during sleep. Sleep walking, night terrors, and tragically, sudden infant death syndrome (SIDS), may be related to sleep dysfunction. But I believe that some of the less dramatic effects of sleep deprivation on children may also prove to be highly destructive.

Bedwetting, for example, while an unpleasant subject at best, appears to be a significant indicator of the quality and quantity of sleep a child is getting. Once again, my research has clearly shown that problems in the sleep cycle are a major factor. Studies show that childhood bedwetters spend too much time in the very deep stages of sleep, probably because they are already physically exhausted. As a result, they are not aware of the signals their bladder is sending when it is full. Instead of awaking, they wet the bed.

In addition, these children experience smaller amounts of REM sleep, the dream state, which is a vital ingredient of healthful sleep and a critical factor in mental stability. During REM sleep, the child's kidneys actually produce less urine than during non-REM sleep. As a result, not only are these children unaware that they need to urinate, they are also producing much larger amounts of urine than children who are sleeping normally. The results are obvious.

I first met Joshua, who was then a bright, but somewhat shy 12 year old, after his mother attended a seminar I gave on premenstrual syndrome. During the seminar, I had mentioned that approximately one-third of the women with incapacitating symptoms of PMS had been late childhood bedwetters. This statistic is particularly impressive when you take into account the fact that only about four percent of children, some 60 percent of them male, continue to wet their beds after the age of seven.

Joshua's mom told me that she too had extremely severe PMS. And that she had wet her bed until the age of 13, only a few weeks before she had her first period. None of this surprised me. When Joshua, her only child, was born she had hoped he would be spared the torment of her own painful childhood. But, as luck would have it, she had married a man who had also been a bedwetter. Since there is certainly a genetic link in these, as well as other brain-chemical conditions (more on this in later chapters), Joshua had the cards stacked against him from birth.

Joshua was already having considerable difficulty in school, and had been singled out by his teachers as a moody, shy, and difficult child. His parents worried that he always seemed tired and often fell asleep in front of the TV and while reading or doing homework.

Extracurricular activities and close friendships were also a problem for Joshua, who always made excuses to avoid overnight trips or parties where his "secret" might be discovered. When he occasionally felt obligated to accept such an invitation, he would stay awake all night in an attempt to avoid wetting his bed.

Of course, Joshua's parents both understood the pain that accompanies this particular malady and were able to handle the situation with considerable sensitivity. However, their sympathy did little to lessen Joshua's discomfort about even discussing the topic. But when I shared my own bedwetting experience with him, he began to open up to me.

Not surprisingly, Joshua's self-image, by this time in his life, was depressingly low. He believed that he was somehow weaker than other children, and that his secret must never be exposed.

The first thing we decided to do was take him off any medication (and his parents had tried a lot of them). I explained that many of his symptoms were caused by the side effects of these drugs, not by his condition. I also let him know that the alarm system which his parents had resorted to in desperation, that sounded when he started to wet his bed, would have to go. He had told me it left him jumpy and wiped out during the day. Joshua, I might add, was relieved to know that he would not have to suffer the tortures of this particular "technological miracle" any longer.

As I had with other bedwetters, I placed Joshua on a two-phase program. The first phase was designed to enhance the brain chemical serotonin through the use of the amino acid L-tryptophan. Unfortunately for Joshua and others like him, this amino acid is no longer available (see Appendix B). The second part of Joshua's program improved the quantity and quality of his sleep (more on this in later chapters). Within a few weeks, Joshua stopped wetting his bed and began to show a marked improvement in disposition. Within a few short months, his teachers began to comment that he was virtually a changed person. Joshua was clearly more positive in outlook, more eager to learn and genuinely happier than anyone could remember. I am happy to report he soon was able to attend the first of many weekend camping trips with his scout troop without worrying about "accidents". Because L-tryptophan is no longer available in the United States, Joshua's parents have been forced to take him to Canada to obtain this vital amino acid. Both Joshua and his parents agree, they are unwilling to give up the many benefits this program has provided.

If bedwetting was just a harmless, however inconvenient, phase that some children must pass through, its relation to sleep problems wouldn't demand much attention. Unfortunately, my research has confirmed an alarmingly high correlation between personal histories of childhood bedwetting and a plethora of behavioral disorders. To begin with, there has been a correlation with children who wet the bed and also either abuse animals or start fires. There is mounting evidence that this behavior in childhood can lead to violent behavior in adulthood.

Later in life, the same children may show a troubling propensity for destructive behavior as adults. Childhood bedwetters may grow up displaying criminal tendencies, alcohol or drug problems, sleep difficulties, depression or mood swings, severe PMS and even suicidal tendencies (more in later chapters). You can often force children to stop wetting the bed by using an alarm system or by depriving them of the deep stages of sleep with drugs, but I maintain that until you treat the underlying brain chemical connection to sleep disorders, these children will continue to have problems.

In the past, childhood bed wetting was generally viewed strictly as an emotional disorder. Children who wet the bed, we were told, were emotionally unstable. Some experts have even suggested that bed wetting is nothing more than a way of getting attention. I'd like to suggest that, in fact, the "acting out" we see in some children stems from a brain-chemical disorder that makes them more emotional because they are already so sleep-deprived. If we can improve children's sleep schedules and enhance the quality of their sleep, I believe we can reap major benefits in terms of their emotional stability and well-being. I also believe that these benefits can extend throughout their adult lives.

As youngsters grow up, their need for slumber gradually decreases, leveling off during the adolescent years. But that doesn't mean that our kids are off the hook. Prior to the onset of puberty, today's children are prey to a wide array of disruptive influences in their immediate surroundings that may mitigate against their ability to sleep. The consequences, I believe, can be seen in the widespread physiological and psychological symptoms currently ascribed to conditions such as learning disabilities, attention-deficit disorders and hyperactivity in children.

Children are not only getting much less sleep than they actually need these days, but the quality of that sleep is often lacking. As a number of pediatricians have come forward in recent years take pains to point out, these disruptive childhood behaviors may be caused by the introduction of artificial ingredients into their diet. Children are subjected to a continuous barrage of advertising for sugar-laden breakfast cereals, soft drinks and snacks in television advertising. And all too often, harried parents comply with their demands for these products, simply to keep the peace.

Extensive research has established that various forms of sugars, sugar substitutes and food additives (colorings, emulsifiers, and preservatives) in packaged foods can play havoc with young metabolisms. Children, especially, appear to be astonishingly susceptible to the biological imbalances that commonly-occurring chemicals in processed foods are known to promote. What amazes me is how reluctant some experts have been to acknowledge the role these adulterants may play in the rising tide of childhood misbehavior. Instead, dubious procedures, such as drugs that act as central nervous system stimulants, continue to be routinely prescribed when there is already plenty of evidence that we can markedly improve these aberrations of behavior simply by improving the child's diet. I would like to suggest that by also improving both the quality and quantity of sleep, a vast improvement in learning and behavior would result.

At the same time, the public's perception regarding artificial ingredients in food such as processed sugar seems to have moved ahead of the medical establishment. Witness the current consumer thrust for products that are low in sugar and calories. Sadly, the answer to the dilemma of avoiding sweets while continuing to crave them has been answered by the food industry with the introduction of a new generation of artificial sweeteners. Interestingly, low brain chemical levels of serotonin also cause sugar cravings (more on this in later chapters).

Artificial sweeteners usually contain active ingredients such as phenylalinine, an amino acid. These sugar substitutes may cause mental and emotional dysfunctions, especially in susceptible children.

While the duration of sleep humans require continues to taper off as we reach puberty, the process may be more gradual than has previously been assumed. As proof, the latest research confirms that as teenagers grow into adolescence, they generally need at least ten and one half hours of sleep every night for optimum performance.

In other words, a teenager who gets up at 7 a.m. each morning has to be in bed, asleep, by 8:30 p.m. to ensure adequate sleep. Given the pressures of homework, household chores and social pursuits to which most teenagers are subjected, it's a safe bet that most of these kids aren't getting the kind of sleep they need. Today's adolescents, therefore, probably constitute the most sleep-deprived age group of all.

Sure enough, surveys show that the typical teenager averages about seven hours of sleep per night, several hours short of the sleep he or she requires. And once again, this usually means being entirely deprived of restorative last-stage REM sleep. As a result, these teenagers have to catch up on their missing sleep either at home on the weekend or, the only other place they can, in the classroom. As serious as the consequences of sleep deprivation for children of school age may be, the phenomenon may have far more serious implications for today's teenagers.

I'll never forget the first time I met Nathan, a sixteen year old whose twin sister Natalie was already my patient. Nathan's parents had sent him to see me when they were virtually at their wits' end. Both teenagers, they felt, were already out of control and headed for trouble.

As it turned out, Natalie suffered from severe mood swings and depression. I had been seeing her in my PMS clinic for about four months. The change in Natalie had already been quite remarkable. Her sleep pattern, once normalized, had begun to turn her into a productive and even, occasionally, cooperative young woman. She felt more rested and had even expressed a sense of well-being that she had never before experienced in her short life.

When Natalie's mother was in with her on a visit, she began to talk with me about the problems they were having with Nathan. After much discussion, I convinced her that both childrens' problems were in fact symptoms of the same disorder. And I agreed to see Nathan, as well.

Nathan had a sullen attitude. He dressed in the latest heavy-metal fashions and had already decided that anything I, or any other adult had to say, was definitely, as he put it, "crap". His grades had been slipping since he had entered junior high school a few years before. Although his parents did not believe Nathan had a serious drug problem, he had spent some time experimenting with marijuana and alcohol. He also spent long hours sulking in his room, listening to the angry music of his favorite heavy-metal bands. Much to his parents' concern, his friends kept him out to all hours of the night and he often skipped school in an attempt to "catch up" on his sleep the next morning. After Nathan had missed classes several times without an appropriate excuse, the school had called his parents in for a conference.

Natalie experienced more severe symptoms than Nathan, and on a cyclic basis, because her menstrual cycle used up more of the important brain chemical, serotonin. Nathan, on the other hand, had more moderate symptoms, but they were more constant. They were worse when he didn't get his sleep, if his diet was poor or if his use of recreational drugs interfered with his sleep.

Although he at first resisted being seen by a woman who was treating PMS, Nathan eventually responded equally well to my program. And once he got over his initial embarrassment and appreciated what I was suggesting, he began to cooperate.

I am delighted to report that both Nathan and Natalie have since graduated from high school and are now attending their last year of college. They pay attention to their sleep, diet, and lifestyle and tell their parents they are feeling great.

When humans are chronically sleep deprived in test situations, they experience periods of what is known as "microsleep", which may last only for a few seconds or for several minutes. Under conditions where subjects may try to assume the appearance of wakefulness, this sleep state may correspond to what we know as daydreaming. I believe that many young students who are categorized with so-called "attention-deficit disorders" are experiencing periods of microsleep throughout the day. And although a microsleep period effectively prevents them from paying attention, they may, in fact, be safeguarding their sanity.

I am firmly convinced that what we are learning about sleep deprivation has enormous implications for our children's learning ability and, ultimately, can tell us much about what's really wrong with our educational system. I've had many teachers tell me that their students routinely fall asleep in class and that when they do stay awake, they have a lot of difficulty concentrating. Either they are daydreaming or they act fatigued. One teacher commented, "It's downright embarrassing to have to wake your students up time and time again in the middle of a lecture."

This problem may be due in part to the nutritional status of many young people. A recent California study suggests that one out of three children in that state goes to bed hungry. It's a safe bet that many more children go to sleep ill-prepared for their nightly sleep cycle by their diet of junk food.

We hear a lot about the failure of our national education system. In this context, I am of the opinion that we are putting the blame in the wrong place. I think society as a whole needs to turn its attention towards ensuring our children get adequate rest in order to ensure they're going to be able to learn effectively. It is not possible for a teacher, no matter how good he or she is, to teach a classroom full of sleep deprived students and expect them to have anything but minimal retention.

If we don't take a long, hard look at this particular issue and how it effects the educational system in this country, we will surely continue to fall behind in all areas of education. Creativity is enhanced through REM sleep or the dreaming state of sleep. If we continue to shorten the sleep cycle and eliminate that critical last phase of REM sleep, we are eliminating our own ability, and that of our children, to experience the creative side of learning.

I would urge policy makers in the school system to start classes an hour later in the morning to accommodate the sleep needs of children. I would also urge teachers to make sleep a high priority in their own lives. We can't expect students to learn if they are being taught by teachers who are themselves sleep deprived. I would further urge parents to make sleep, nutrition and a stable, loving family high priorities in their lives.

There's another, darker side to the phenomenon of teen sleep deprivation. I believe there may be a connection between poor sleep and the dramatic rise in the incidence of suicide among this age group in recent years. According to the Center for Disease Control the suicide rate for teens has quadrupled over the past forty years. Experts have blamed this self-destructive epidemic on everything from broken homes and "copy-cat" behavior to purported satanic messages in heavy metal rock music.

Here again, I think that, instead, the finger points to sleep deprivation as a decisive factor in teenage disorientation, depression and violence. Teenagers who miss several hours of sleep every night of the week, like other sleep-deprived subjects in human tests, will tend to be especially suggestible to negative messages. Kids who are sleep deprived and already under heavy stress from peer pressure and the insecurities of adolescence, and who are then exposed to self-destructive suggestions in rock lyrics, may in fact be victims of brainwashing at a subconscious level. In addition, we also have the high incidence of drugs and alcohol, which further disrupt the sleep cycle and cause changes in mood and behavior.

In other words, parents who think they can solve the problems of teen suicide, alcohol and drug abuse or depression with simple "just say no" campaigns are missing the point. Parents, in my opinion, would be better off to see that their children are well rested and mentally alert. In turn, these children would be capable of making more rational decisions in their daily lives. This is going to be extremely difficult to get across since most parents are severely sleep-deprived themselves.

As we grow to adulthood, the amount of sleep we require continues to decrease gradually (although perhaps not as much as we would like to believe). Most people think they need approximately eight hours of sleep when they reach their twenties. I think that nine-plus hours of sleep per night is necessary for most people, and that we simply get used to less sleep in response to the heavy demands on wakefulness experienced by young parents and people who are just starting out in their careers. After all, as I've said before, humans really haven't changed a bit, from a physiological point of view, since the invention of the light bulb when our ancestors were still sleeping nine to ten hours per night.

As we approach middle age, the amount of sleep we need does not diminish. We simply don't sleep as well when we grow older. By age 50, the national sleep average is down to about six hours per night. And by age 70, significantly less than six hours is the norm. But the fact that older people often sleep less, probably has more to do with the physical infirmities of age than any inherent lack of, or need for, sleep. Whether due to pain, illness, medication or incontinence, sleep interruptions are known to increase dramatically in later years (as shown by the higher incidence of sleep disorders among the elderly).

Lack of sleep, in turn, tends to aggravate the symptoms of old age, sometimes making illness worse and contributing to states of frustration, confusion and depression. Paradoxically, at the time in their lives when most people can look forward to unlimited rest and relaxation, their ability to do so is in decline.

As in other age groups, our society's ingrained bias against sleep tends to work against the welfare of the elderly. Adult children who care for their parents often find themselves confronted with the problem of an elderly mother or father who in many ways places the same demands on their time and energy as an infant. In turn, friends and doctors often support them in rejecting or down-playing their parents' complaints about sleep problems.

These complaints grow more frequent as people continue to age. By and large, elderly sleep distress involves nighttime arousal and its counterpart, daytime sleepiness. While approximately one third of Americans report sleep problems, more than half of people over the age of 65 have the same complaint. Not surprisingly, the elderly, although they make up no more than 15 percent of the population, purchase twice as many prescriptions for nighttime sedatives as the rest of us. Or about 30 percent of sleeping pills consumed.

An important clue to people's increasing inability to sleep with age is found in their internal clock, also known as Circadian rhythms. These rhythms tend to go out of synch in the brains of older people. This, in turn, creates a tendency in the elderly to have difficulty sleeping at night, along with daytime sleepiness. We have all seen older folks nodding off in their chairs. If elderly people do not get adequate, quality nighttime sleep, they will often drop off to sleep as soon as they relax during the day. It has also been shown that a person's proportion of dreaming (REM) sleep and deep (non-REM) sleep periods undergoes a significant shift with the passage of time. All these factors combine to contribute to the familiar experience among older people of increased nighttime wakefulness, less deep sleep, more shallow sleep, and awaking earlier, feeling as though they hadn't slept at all.

2 Generation Gaps

Theodore was a 70 year old man who had begun to experience some changes in his memory. He often found himself walking along a street and was unable to remember where he was going or, in fact, where he had been. He was beginning to worry. As he indicated in our first meeting, "Perhaps I have Alzheimer's disease or maybe I'm just getting old."

Theodore was also having a lot of daytime drowsiness. He often was found asleep, just napping in his chair by his wife. She was also beginning to be concerned about his behavior. She told me that over the past several years, he had begun to be very irritable and sometimes snapped at her, arguing over the most insignificant things. Theodore had begun to take tranquilizers about 10 years before for insomnia. Prior to his retirement, he had been an executive who commanded the respect of many people under him. He was accustomed to making high-powered decisions and exercising his mind on a regular basis. Around the time retirement became eminent, he began to experience some periods of anxiety and some periods of sleeplessness. His doctor prescribed tranquilizers (benzodiazipines) to ease his anxiety. As the retirement progressed and he spent more time at home, he became more depressed and more irritable. His doctor had, therefore, increased the amount of the tranquilizer he was taking. In addition, he had been prescribed medications to treat his high blood pressure. The change in his personality, according to his wife, had been a gradual one. One that had gotten persistently worse as time passed. Prior to this, his wife confided, they had been happily married for over 40 years. Now, however, Theodore was getting more and more difficult to live with every day.

Theodore was very worried about his health. He no longer felt happiness or joy and he attributed this to his recent retirement. After meeting with Theodore and his wife, I first performed a medical history and a thorough physical examination with all the appropriate laboratory work. I then consulted with his physician regarding the use of his tranquilizers. We determined that Theodore would be tapered off of his medications gradually and that a program of serotonin enhancement and sleep hygiene was indicated.

Theodore's recovery was absolutely remarkable. He began to experience a gradual increase in mood in a very short time. In a matter of weeks, he began to feel more cheerful and he noticed that his memory was returning. He was also feeling much more alert during the day. He continues to take naps in the afternoon, and he continues to sleep better at night. He also began a gradual program of stress reduction exercise and some dietary modifications. We felt this would be appropriate for, not only his sleep hygiene, but also his other medical problems.

I'm happy to report that Theodore is now a 75 year old, active, committed member of society. He has started working with an entrepreneurial program which pairs retired executives with young entrepreneurs, and he feels that he is making a vital contribution to this program. He's walking daily, feeling more vigor than he has in years. His wife also reports a significant change in Theodore and also claims that, by helping her husband, she also helped herself. She, too, is feeling better than she has in years.

It should be clear by now that the amount of sleep we need during our lives changes dramatically from infancy to old age. And while subtle changes in the kind of sleep we need at various times in our lives also play a part in the quality of our sleep, we all have the same basic sleep requirements. It is equally true that all too often, we fail to fulfill our requirements for healthful sleep. All the same, I'm convinced that there is much you can do to adapt to our changing needs for sleep. You can take control of your own sleep patterns and teach your family to do the same—sleep matters.

The following is a sleep schedule according to age.

Newborns:	16-18 hours per day.
Age 1-5:	13-14 hours per day.
Age 6-12:	12-13 hours per day.
Age 13-18:	10-11 hours per day.
Young Adults:	9-10 hours per day.
Middle Age:	8-10 hours per day.
Seniors:	8-10 hours per day.

3 Asleep on the Job

Crisis in the Workplace

Z Z Z Z Z Z Z Z Z Z Z Z Z Z Z Z Z Z Z Z Z Z Z Z Z

We've already seen how society is affected by our collective sleep debt. We've also seen how negative attitudes towards sleep can affect our quality of life at every age. By the same token, the costs of sleep loss in terms of human pain and suffering are equally evident when America goes to work.

Every Sunday morning when the weekend newspaper arrives on the doorstep, readers across the country are treated to another installment in the humorous misadventures of Dagwood Bumstead. The hapless hero of Blondie, as just about any recent episode will confirm, is obviously a victim of chronic sleep deprivation. When he's not working far into the night to finish some complicated report for his domineering boss, Dagwood is sleeping late and forgetting his briefcase (or his pants) in his mad rush to get to work. On weekends, he's still a basket case and his unfinished projects around the house always seem to end with a nap on the living room couch.

It doesn't require a great stretch of the imagination to connect the popularity of Blondie with our collective insecurities where the subject of sleep is concerned. But unlike the situations Dagwood faces on the comics page, the reality of sleep loss, for most working Americans anyway, is far from amusing.

Sleep loss manifests itself first, even before we arrive at work. A growing body of research confirms what many experts have suspected all along, namely that inadequate sleep, even if it's as little as an hour or two less than usual, can significantly increase the chances of human error. And the times we need sleep the most are often exactly the same times at which most of us aren't getting it.

This is especially true during two peak periods when the urge to sleep is at its strongest. These periods have been identified in experiments as the times when subjects were most likely to lapse into inadvertent sleep episodes. The first period comes during the early hours of the morning (about 4 to 6 am), about the time when most people are being awakened by their alarm clocks, and again, though to a lesser extent, during the late afternoon. Sure enough, motorists who fall asleep at the wheel in traffic follow the same two-peak pattern, a major one in the early morning hours and another in mid-afternoon. Unfortunately, this is also when many of us are driving to our jobs and, coincidentally, traffic accidents happen most often at these times.

Eerily enough, human mortality rates are correlated with the same familiar two-peak pattern. No doubt this is partly related to the accident figures, but more probably because physiological processes associated with mortality coincide with the chemistry of sleep.

As a society, we're only now discovering how much impact sleep-related processes can have in a whole range of major workplace disasters, from Chernobyl to the space shuttle, and in a myriad of lesser tragedies ranging from airplane crashes to fatal miscalculations and equipment malfunctions.

It is also becoming apparent that sleep deprivation affects people more profoundly than we realize, in ways that could have far-reaching implications for our national interest. Studies show that missing out on certain critical periods of sleep can have insidious side effects, although the damage may not be especially noticeable even when sleep loss is habitual.

In experiments, human subjects who were sleep deprived were found to perform routine functions with no noticeable lack of skill. Only when they were faced with making creative decisions did the effects of sleep deprivation become noticeable. Sleep deprived subjects failed miserably when it came to making decisions that depended on cognitive skills. Chronically sleep-deprived people suffer most in the morning, when they have more trouble thinking analytically. Loss of sleep during the final hours of the sleep cycle was found to be especially significant in this regard (more on this in later chapters).

Workers who are roused from bed before they are finished sleeping can, therefore, be expected to be less capable of creative problem-solving, which is often called for when making split-second decisions. By mid-day, the sleep deprived appear to recover their faculties, scoring as well on cognitive tests as their better-rested counterparts. By that time, however, the damage has been done.

This brings us to one of the most debilitating aspects of chronic sleep deprivation. It's a kind of self-fulfilling prophecy. In other words, if you know you haven't been getting enough sleep, you're going to be stressed out about trying to get more. Unfortunately, the more intent you are on going to sleep, the harder it will be to drift off. Experts refer to a chronically sleep-deprived person's anguished anticipation of bedtime as "learned insomnia".

Psychologists warn that the chronically sleep-deprived also tend to be far more vulnerable to depression and anxiety than those who get their rest. They tend to be overly concerned about health problems as well. If you're not getting enough sleep, you may be prone to a condition known as "depressed pessimism". Losing sleep can leave you with a negative outlook on life that may be at odds with reality. Often physiologically induced, it's what's likely to make you feel incompetent about the job you're doing even though you're working as well as ever. It seems possible that America's poor sleep habits are also reflected in the soaring rates of absenteeism seen in industry, as well as on-the-job injuries and accidents. Victims of sleep deprivation will also experience significantly increased stress, because they don't feel up to their jobs.

Psychological stress tests focus on these same symptoms of sleep loss, and workers' stress levels are gauged according to their subjective impression of the quality of their jobs. I don't think it's a coincidence that complaints about job stress now amount to roughly 10 percent of all occupational disease claims. Ten years ago, stress claims were just about zero. While this may in part be due to an increased awareness of the physiological role of stress, the same figures seem to argue for an escalating pattern of sleep loss in modern society. Interestingly, from 1969 to 1989 the average work load has increased by 158 hours per year. This is equal to one extra month of work a year. Add to this the fact that from 1981 to 1989 leisure time has decreased by 15% and you can see that society is getting pretty tired.

Once again, society's sleep macho attitude works in favor of those whose genes or conditioning allow them to get by with less sleep. At least one prominent researcher has claimed that subjects who get less than the bare minimum of sleep each night, and don't need more to feel wide awake, are often more energetic, efficient, and unworried than normal.

By contrast, according to experts, subjects who require more than nine hours sleep tend to be more introspective, fretful people. I wonder if these studies don't reflect a kind of chicken-and-egg mentality. In other words, which comes first, a predisposition to moodiness, or a need to get more sleep? Here again, the cards are stacked against those who need more sleep.

One of the most radical changes to have taken place in recent years concerns the increasing numbers of married women in the work force. You may have noticed that even Blondie herself, the long-suffering homemaker of the comic strips, has joined the ranks of working mothers. We've already seen how most women probably need more sleep than their mates and also, how the time of night when they feel ready to sleep often works to their disadvantage. Working at a steady job only serves to compound the problem.

Another aspect of sleep deprivation that is only now being understood is the impact of nighttime arousals on the overall quality of sleep. Studies show that daytime function is affected by the continuity, as well as by the amount of sleep. And obviously nighttime arousals are a big factor for working mothers with young children.

Studies show that women with careers actually sleep about five percent less each night than men with similar job demands which adds to the female burden of sleep loss. Perhaps because of some innate biological sense that they already aren't getting enough sleep, women appear to sacrifice what's called "nonmarket time" (time not spent on the job) to make up for this percentage, while men routinely cut the actual hours of sleep they need. The real irony here is that women actually require at least one hour more sleep than do men.

But that may be too simple, especially when we consider that most working women are still expected to shoulder the double burden of child-rearing and domestic duties. A working husband might cut back on his sleep, but he can afford to spend much of his time away from work in leisure activities and relaxation, a luxury that is denied most working wives. These women must understand intuitively that they simply can't afford to lose sleep when virtually every waking hour is devoted to work of some form or other.

I met Alice after a seminar I had given on premenstrual syndrome. Alice was a 42 year old executive who had three children. Two of her children were almost grown, ages 17 and 19, and the third was age three. After the birth of her youngest, she noticed a marked increase in fatigue, irritability and depression. Over the next three years, she sought the advise of several doctors, counselors, chiropractors, and even tried herbal therapy and acupuncture. But she had never had anything but the most minimal relief from her symptoms. Alice continued to work 60 to 70 hours per week and confided in me, "I still feel that the housework and childcare is primarily my responsibility."

Because her husband and children showed little patience or understanding for her problems, the pressure mounted. Her husband belittled the whole situation, and summed it up by saying, "I've just got one of those women who bitches." Her children and other family members accused her of deliberately dramatizing the situation. Each family member felt they were contributing equally. In addition to her career, Alice also volunteered outside the home and was involved in community work. If her children needed a parent volunteer, they always suggested their mother. Needless to say, Alice had little time left over for sleep.

She became increasingly withdrawn from family and friends. She argued frequently with family members over trivial matters. This behavior was so totally unlike her natural self that she began to have very real fears for her sanity.

During her first consultation with me, it became clear she was extremely sleep deprived and suffering from superwoman syndrome. I told her I had recently heard on a talk show that superwoman was dead; she died of exhaustion! This brought the first hint of a smile I had seen since she entered my office. After Alice started on my program, she improved steadily. In addition to the sleep hygiene and serotonin enhancement, we enlisted her family in the household duties and sought creative solutions to time management.

At present she is working 50 hours a week, but says she is so much more efficient. She is accomplishing more than she did when working 60 to 70 hours each week. She has a part-time housekeeper, and the family has pitched in to help. She sleeps much better and wakes up feeling rested and refreshed, and she adds, "I think my family is even happier than I am to have the old me back."

From all this, it's evident that we need to be far more concerned about the impact of sleep loss on the workplace. Take the phenomenon of "fast-track" careers, for example. Studies have even established a correlation between higher incomes and sleep loss. Researchers have shown that a 25 percent wage increase reduces sleep time by about ten minutes per night. The men and women who are in decision-making positions are actually less well rested than the people who work for them.

Most of the major advances that have happened in the workplace have come about by utilizing the 80 or 90 percent of our brain power which is our unconscious or creative side, as opposed to using the 10 to 20 percent brain power which is logical thinking. When one begins to realize the impact that losing sleep can have on our future and the economic future of this country, we begin to see the high price being paid for sleep loss. Creative solutions to problems which face the everyday man, as well as executives, become elusive, and we begin to fall further and further behind in the world economy. Americans have long been known for their inventiveness, and, until recently, this has been a driving force in our economic growth. Executives and workers alike need to have some choices in their sleep schedules if we are to remain a leader in new ideas.

Part of the job stress is undoubtedly influenced by recent economic trends. As stated earlier, the American economy is in trouble, and the recent downturn is often blamed on our increasing inability to maintain a technological edge. Of course, we've seen how sleep loss may have a lot to do with that, as well. For the most part, American workers are over-worked and seriously sleep deprived.

Economists will tell you when you work at 100% of capacity productivity actually decreases. Industry, however, has failed to see the disastrous consequences of downsizing. This is the term used to describe how industry is dealing with the new economic realities, and many observers view the trend with alarm. Those who stay on the job are working longer hours. Along with the insecurity that comes with the restructuring and reducing of corporate ranks, psychologists see workers' problems with depression and anxiety manifested in a greater incidence of suicide, alcoholism, drug abuse and domestic violence. And, I believe if the trend continues, this situation will only escalate.

The last decade of salary cuts, plant closures and early retirement has pretty much backed America's labor force into a financial corner. Statistics show that among new openings in the U.S. job market, more than half of them pay less than the poverty level for a family of four. It's not surprising that approximately one in twelve American workers now hold two, or more jobs, or that more women are going to work. And for many of them, men, as well as women, that means working shifts.

As I noted in the introduction to this book, there is plenty of historical evidence showing that, up until a century ago, people slept an average of nine and a half hours per night, hours more than we do now. Back in the late 1800's, when Thomas Edison's most famous invention changed our sleeping habits forever, another social upheaval was taking place in the factory. This is where the introduction of electric light had its first major impact. Just as the light bulb pushed back the natural boundaries of wake and sleep, so the same technological innovation created a highly lucrative option for industry. When the lights stayed on, as early capitalists quickly realized, there was no need to shut down. Factories and service industries could function virtually around the clock, creating immense profits for their owners.

What the industry barons didn't fully appreciate was the human toll that shift work takes. Knowing what we do now about inattention from lack of sleep, it's obvious that unnatural wake and sleep periods have the potential for disaster. The problem is compounded by the fact that most people who work nights are often in positions where a great deal depends on making "snap decisions" with relatively little supervision or contact with co-workers.

While most adults today are steadily employed, the way we work is differentiated in significant ways by when we work. For example, if you're typical, you probably arrive for work around eight o'clock in the morning and leave around five o'clock in the afternoon. This schedule is as old as time itself. It's governed by the archetypal cycle of wake and sleep.

Many of us, however, punch a different clock. Today, shift work is an unavoidable fact of life in the workplace. According to surveys, approximately one out of four American males (and one out of six women) are employed in shift work. From the people who pilot that late-night flight you're coming in on, to the ones who process your overnight bank transfers or those who are responsible for your nightly safety and protection, more and more Americans are being forced to get by on very little of the right kind of sleep.

Small wonder many sleep-deprived workers are known to resort to alcohol or drugs as a means of compensating for fatigue. In that regard, perhaps we should think about redirecting some of the enormous investment of time and energy involved in testing workers for drugs, with the difficult questions of privacy and constitutional freedoms that entails, to insuring that workers get the sleep they need.

It's not just about putting in long hours or not getting enough rest, although that's bad enough. What happens is men and women who work evening and night shifts have to absorb a kind of one-two punch. The one-fifth of salaried workers in our country who are in this category are routinely required to rotate their hours of labor through day, evening or night duty, according to obsolete stereotypes which are at odds with what we now know about wake and sleep.

Not only are shift workers routinely unable to sleep when they should, worse, conventional shift-work schedules are hopelessly unrealistic in terms of people's ability to compensate for forced changes in their wake/sleep patterns. Deprived of natural sleep, nighttime workers are desynchronized from their sleep/wake cycle.

You'd expect that there might have been some fine-tuning in recent years of the sleep/wake schedule we assign to the significant proportion of the work force who toil at night. In fact, it isn't so. Modern day shift-work is dictated by the same time clock established, coincidentally, with the invention of the lightbulb more than one hundred years ago.

The guidelines for shift work, as laid down in the late 1800's during the heyday of the Industrial Revolution were, and by and large still are, that you work one shift for five straight days, then get two days off to recuperate, then switch shifts, and so forth. Presumably, this schedule was devised in a misguided spirit of fairness, that is, in this way no one has to work nights more than anyone else.

The problem is that this staggered work schedule doesn't help even remotely to allow shift workers to function at peak efficiency. And while some employers have experimented with more realistic schedules designed to minimize disruption of innate sleep rhythms, by and large our guidelines for shift work belong where they began, back in the 19th century.

Disruption of normal sleep schedules aside, the problem of sleep deprivation is particularly acute when workers are chronically deprived of sleep as part of their job activity. Medical school graduates, for example, are required to complete their education as residents in hospitals. While there's been plenty of criticism of this system which mandates 30 to 60 hour continuous shifts and tours of duty from 90 to 130 hours per week (in other words, 12 to 18 hour work days), for the unfortunate recruits, little has been done to change the status quo.

As a result, for most patients admitted to the care of their local hospital staff, chances are good that treatment is being administered by some over-worked, acutely sleep-deprived, medical school graduate, assisted by an equally overworked and acutely, sleep deprived nurse. As a matter of fact, there was a case where a severely fatigued resi-dent was performing surgery when he actually fell asleep on his patient. This is not the kind of quality performance most of us would hope for. Chances of physician error have greatly increased because technological advances now allow critically ill patients to survive longer. But at the same time, this technology requires more complex clinical judgements based on relatively imperceptible subtleties of a patient's condition. And while rational and biologically sound limits to hospital staff work hours are commonplace in other industrialized countries and have been leg-islated in some states, economic concerns about these changes have slowed the pace of change. This is due primarily to pressure from national and state medical societies.

Nighttime employees who are responsible for industrial safety are in a critical enough position where sleep loss is concerned, as we know from investigations of everything from nuclear reactor accidents to plane crashes. But an even subtler and more pervasive dynamic comes into play when decision-making involves so-called "judgement calls". For instance, you probably wouldn't want someone who is chronically sleep-deprived holding a gun on you in a tense confrontation, but that's exactly what happens with many police officers in the line of duty. It's no accident that recently the media has seen a rash of what is termed "police brutality". Many of these officers have themselves been the victims of a system that forces them to work in a sleep deprived state. I'm sure you'll agree that policemen and policewomen perform a vital function in our society. Unfortunately, they're also frequently victimized by cavalier attitudes regarding when and how they should sleep.

Police work may be one of the most vulnerable occupations where sleep loss is concerned. True to their macho image, officers pride themselves on being able to perform at peak efficiency at any hour of the day or night, and we expect them to live up to that. But when the discrepancy between the sleep they need and the sleep they get is acute, then mishaps, even fatal ones, can easily happen.

Worse still, such individuals are discouraged from dealing with obvious symptoms of sleep loss, even when they suspect that their disruptive work schedules may be to blame for their problems. For example, I know of one career police officer who had been working the night shift in a neighboring community for the last several years. After being reassigned to the day shift, he returned to his regular night shift after only a few short weeks. That brief respite, as it turned out, had serious physical and mental repercussions.

This officer was now in a double bind because he sensed that he couldn't let his superiors know about the emotional turmoil he was experiencing. He felt compelled to discuss the situation with his station chief because no one else had been of help in changing his shift. At the same time, he feared that such a discussion would show up in his personnel file. Then he would be branded as a "weak" person in need of psychological counselling, all because of the extreme burnout and difficulty with sleep he had to report. I can only wonder, how many other police workers suffer the same unbearable stresses in their jobs, and whether these pressures aren't to blame, in many ways, for some of the outrageous outbreaks of police brutality we see in the news these days.

If this all sounds pretty hopeless, remember that creative solutions abound for the problems I've described. Schedules, for example, that allow workers to stay home for three or four days a week need to be looked at more carefully. While they have the potential for abuse, working longer hours on the days they are at their jobs isn't exactly what the doctor ordered. It seems to me that the drawbacks outweigh the benefits of this particular solution. Workers who can spend more "quality time" with their families and who have more nights in a row to catch up on sleep should be able to handle longer work days far more easily. Most employers pay a shift differential for working graveyard or swing shifts. I think a better solution might be to work fewer hours, with longer recovery time for these shift workers. And frankly, I think society needs to take a look at how important some of these night shifts really are. Obviously, emergency personnel need to be available 24 hours a day. But, is it really necessary to grocery shop at 4:00 a.m?

Employers also need to begin to look at the importance of providing flex time for their workers. If significant portions of the work force were going to their jobs a bit earlier or a bit later, we would not only see an improvement in congestion during rush hours, we would also be sparing employees the extra stress of navigating in hectic traffic conditions. If workers were allowed to take longer lunch hours, afternoon naps might become a viable option. I'll probably be kidded for this, but as a firm believer in the value of naps, I'd like to see progressive firms set up nap rooms for their overworked staffs. Or perhaps organize work schedules, so mid-shift breaks occur in the hours of late afternoon when more of us are likely to take advantage of the need for sleep. Another creative solution is to allow some employees to work out of their homes.

One pressing problem of sleep deprivation for the work force that is being dealt with more creatively these days concerns the popular phenomenon of jet lag. Most airline passengers are travelling on business, and so, when their itineraries involve long, transcontinental flights, we can expect that to impact job performance. Fortunately, there is plenty of information about ways to mitigate the effects of jet lag. Later, I will make some suggestions that are probably new to you about overcoming this unhappy fact of modern life.

Next, we'll consider some of the most tragic consequences of chronic sleep deprivation for society, but not before I repeat that, if we are going to avert the sleep crisis in America's workplace, we have to drastically redefine our priorities where sleep is concerned. If we do, I believe we can reap the benefits of better sleep in ways we can now only imagine—sleep matters!

4 *Night Terrors*

The Dark Side of Sleep Debt

Z Z Z Z Z Z Z Z Z Z Z Z Z Z Z Z Z Z Z Z Z Z Z Z

Up to now, this discussion of sleep has been primarily concerned with chronic sleep deprivation. That is, where sleeplessness persists over a long period of time. But what happens to our mental outlook when chronic sleep deprivation becomes acute, and its symptoms are particularly severe?

If it's true that many of us aren't getting enough of the kind of sleep we need, it's also true that some of us don't get any proper sleep at all. Acute sleep deprivation, we are now realizing, has consequences for all sorts of modern day problems in this country, from escalating rates of recidivism among prison inmates to the catastrophic statistics of homeless persons.

These problems aren't just confined to society's outcasts either. For far too many people, a good night's sleep isn't an option. It's an impossibility. For them, sleep deprivation is the sole determining factor in every aspect of their daily lives. The victims include the mentally ill, people with immune problems, those who suffer from unremitting pain and a variety of other sleepless human beings who are routinely discriminated against and ostracized because the true nature of their problem is poorly understood.

Perhaps, it would be more accurate to describe these severe sleepless states many unfortunate people suffer as both chronic and acute. That is to say, what happens when someone is severely sleep deprived, but over a long period of time? Studies of sleep loss have tended to focus on marathon experiments where sleep or dream deprivation is absolute, but of brief duration. Very little attention has been paid to the consequences of prolonged, extreme, partial, sleep deprivation which I believe is at the root of a broad spectrum of societal ills.

What's particularly frightening about all this is how easily any of us can succumb. Severe sleep problems are not restricted to society's misfits. In a sense, chronic, acute sleep deprivation is a hole that anybody can fall into. Experts use the term clinical sleep disorders to describe what happens when sleeplessness becomes a matter of medical concern. While I would argue that all sleep disorders should be taken into account by doctors. I am gratified that medical experts seem to be paying better attention to severe sleep disorders, and perhaps more important, that medicine has begun to recognize that many physical and emotional problems are associated with sleeplessness or a poor quality of sleep.

The most commonly recognized sleep complaint is, of course, insomnia which is estimated to affect one out of three American adults. Unlike more dramatic forms of sleep deprivation, it doesn't take much to get the insomnia ball rolling. The day after effects of stress-induced insomnia tend to overflow to the next night. At this point, insomnia itself is now the source of stress. The sufferer lies in bed worrying about whether he or she will catch up on missing sleep, all of which stimulates a built-in arousal system and makes it that much harder to doze off and then sleep soundly.

In addition, the sleep of an estimated 60 million Americans, not to mention their spouses, is disrupted each night by snoring. The problem is particularly acute for the elderly. (Probably because people tend to gain weight as they age and the extra fatty tissue they build up, especially in the nose and throat, may make it more difficult to breathe while sleeping.) In addition, a brain chemical, serotonin, which is critical for normal sleep also declines with age. Women, furthermore, are much more likely to suffer insomnia than men, and this is partially due to the fact that the menstrual cycle in women causes a decline in serotonin levels. By the age of 60, an estimated 65 percent of men and 40 percent of women snore with over half exhibiting to some extent what is known as "sleep apnea," a condition where the sufferer actually stops breathing for anywhere from 10 seconds to three minutes. In extreme cases, sleep apneas can occur hundreds of times a night.

All in all, roughly 85 sleep disorders have been identified to date, ranging from sleep walking to such "bizarre" sleep disorders as parasomnias (where sleepers act out aggressive or violent behavior), bedwetting or even eating or driving while asleep.

While it's risky to speculate about the root causes of severe sleep disorders, I've come to the conclusion that one clue to the sleeplessness epidemic may lie in a certain neuroendocrine dysfunction which affects many people and which is probably hereditary in nature. This disruption of metabolism may predispose certain people to chronic sleep problems later in life. Childhood bedwetting, sleep walking, night terrors and insomnia may serve as warning signals alerting us to all sorts of behavioral irregularities.

Largely unrecognized as a sleep disorder is premenstrual syndrome (PMS) which was the subject of my first book, *THE PRE-MENSTRUAL SOLUTION, How to Tame the Shrew in You*, Arrow Press, 1987. This sleep disorder affects 60 million American women. But this condition is not just limited to PMS. Women who suffer from postpartum depression are also suffering from a severe form of sleep deprivation. It doesn't take a brain surgeon to figure out that new mothers are, in fact, one of the most sleep deprived groups of people around. Just ask anyone who has stayed up a few nights with a new baby. Because women require more sleep than men and few of them are actually sleeping longer, they are at higher risk to develop other associated sleep problems.

Depression can, of course, affect men and women. Severe depression can change a person's entire perception of their life and surroundings. It isn't really surprising to note that statistically more women suffer from depression than do their male counterparts. The reasons for this are two-fold. First, as I stated earlier, women have lower levels of serotonin at least during the second half of their menstrual cycles. And, second, women generally require one additional hour of sleep per night than men. These people have biological depression in much the same way as certain people suffer from biological diabetes.

In fact, chronic sleep deprivation appears to be one of the most critical factors in modulation of human emotional stability. A person's attitude may be completely controlled by sleep or lack of it. An impressive number of studies have established that test subjects deprived of normal sleep develop symptoms of irritability, depression, mental confusion, rage and even psychotic behavior. We all feel some of these symptoms from time to time. However, when these feelings escalate people may be driven to suicide or homicide simply because they were not getting the sleep they so desperately needed. I don't think it's an accident that with the decrease in the number of hours people sleep each night, there has been an increase in domestic violence.

The realities of chronic sleep deprivation became painfully obvious to me during research I conducted in the prison system. One of the first people I interviewed was a female inmate whom I'll call Carla. Jailed for inciting a drunken brawl and attacking a policeman, Carla had a long history of violent episodes and alcoholic behavior dating back to her early teens. But, as I talked with her, I began to realize that behind the facade of violence and alcoholic behavior, I was seeing an intelligent, articulate and, actually, quite likeable woman.

As Carla opened up to me, she recounted a childhood fraught with episodes of violence from abusive, alcoholic parents, and punctuated by regular nightly incidents involving yelling and beatings at the hands of her father. It was obvious that Carla had spent much of her childhood never knowing when the next eruption of domestic violence would occur. She could recall having persistent problems with nightmares and childhood night terrors over the years, compounding her fears to the point where she told me she felt afraid to even fall asleep at night.

Sure enough, I noticed tell-tale dark circles under Carla's eyes. And her general appearance was one of extreme fatigue. Whatever role her ravaged sleep patterns may have played in Carla's subsequent behavior problems, her condition was clearly not improved by being trapped in the prison environment. I eventually was forced to conclude that it wasn't confinement alone that was provoking the feelings of hostility and depression Carla complained about so bitterly.

These symptoms, I believe, were not necessarily caused solely by her incarceration, but primarily by the fact that Carla, like other inmates, was exposed to conditions that made getting a good night's sleep impossible. While other factors might enter into the equation, Carla complained it was too cold for her to sleep at night and that the air quality inside the prison was extremely poor. Overcrowded prisons are horribly, noisy places, day or night. And any peace and quiet an inmate can get is repeatedly shattered at all hours by the sounds of heated arguments, clanging metal bars and the pounding of footsteps on concrete.

Furthermore, because the lights were kept burning brightly all night for security purposes, Carla's chances of getting a good night's sleep were brutally curtailed. Either from boredom of confinement or because of general exhaustion, Carla, like most inmates, dozed fitfully on and off during the day in irregular sleep patterns. Small wonder, Carla told me she actually felt worse in prison than she did on the outside.

Fortunately, after Carla's release I was able to help Carla by teaching her techniques to improve her sleep. She now holds a full-time job, has been sober for over two years, and no longer exhibits the abusive, violent behavior that led to her incarceration. In fact, Carla tells me now for the first time in her life she feels real hope, real joy and a deep sense of happiness, something she had never experienced in the past.

While Carla's recovery was extremely gratifying to me, I believe her predicament pinpoints one of the gravest problems with our prison system. I also believe that by improving the sleep environment both inside and outside prisons, society could dramatically decrease the incidence of criminal and violent behavior.

The plight of the homeless can similarly be viewed as another exercise in chronic sleep deprivation. Homeless people, whether living on the street or in city shelters, experience many of the same terrible sleeping conditions that inmates do in prisons. Whether sleeping indoors or out, a homeless person who isn't mentally disoriented to begin with, soon will be. Cold, noise, bright lights complicated by the fear of assault or robbery by other street denizens and the necessity to keep moving, will quickly play havoc with whatever healthy sleep patterns he or she has managed to retain. Thus, begins a downward spiral that is nearly impossible to break.

The grim fact is that many homeless people are already sleep deprived in insidious and devastating ways. I believe it is of significant interest that so many of today's homeless are Vietnam veterans (some estimates place the proportion of Vietnam vets as high as 30 to 40 percent). It could be that the symptoms of post-traumatic stress syndrome which continue to afflict so many of our returning soldiers are, in fact, rooted in sleep deprivation.

While there seems to have been little research on the subject in the post-Vietnam era, a review of clinical literature from World War II, the Korean War and the1973 Arab-Israeli War indicates that combat stress casualties were almost always associated with sleep deprivation. The reality of this painful situation was brought vividly home to me by the experiences of an ex-serviceman who was one of my patients.

Monroe was 42 years old when I first met him. A married man with a loving wife, a nice home and three children, he was clearly suffering from post-traumatic stress syndrome. In fact, he was pretty much at the end of his rope. He had been to see many counselors, and had participated in veterans' support groups. And although he felt these activities helped a bit, he was tormented by intense nightmares involving the horrors of war he had witnessed while on tours of duty in Vietnam.

In one recurrent nightmare, Monroe found himself fighting off the enemy while surrounded hour after hour. By the end of the dream, he was always the last person left alive, still shooting, maiming and killing his attackers as quickly as he could in a desperate frenzy. During these episodes, he often jumped up from the bed, grabbed his wife around the neck and tried to strangle her. At other times, he landed on the floor, crouching in a corner. Needless to say, Monroe always awoke from this nightmare feeling completely exhausted.

In what I feel was a revealing parallel to Carla's situation, Monroe also had a childhood history of sleep problems. Always a light sleeper, he remembered being bothered by general fatigue long before he entered the military. He also admitted he had been a bedwetter until he was twelve years old.

Understandably, Monroe's nighttime behavior was taking its toll on his wife, as well. And his inner torment had started to spill over into his relations in the outside world. He found himself getting into physical combative situations with people over even slight disagreements. Often, he found himself confusing his interactions with an impulse to kill his perceived enemies.

Naturally, I was extremely interested by Monroe's accounts of his nighttime experiences in Vietnam, and how, while in the infantry, he had endured many successive days and nights of little or no sleep, constantly on alert. He remembered dozing off at these times for up to an hour. In this, of course, Monroe wasn't alone. Ground troops in Vietnam were exposed to punishing regimens and chronically deprived of sleep. I wasn't surprised when Monroe stated, as a well-known fact, that virtually all of the infantrymen he knew were taking amphetamines to stay awake.

Monroe's experience fits in well with what we know about the effects of even brief periods of sleep deprivation. We know that subjects accrue about a 25 percent drop in their ability to think, plan and execute with every 24 consecutive hours in which they are kept awake. After 72 hours without sleep, subjects' ability to function cognitively is reduced by 75 percent. And when sleep comes in snatches, it does not come without cost. Fragmented sleep may not be sufficiently recuperative. Many experts believe, once again as I noted earlier in this book, the body can do with just rest, but the brain desperately needs sleep.

Research has shown that a transient, stressful situation of the kind Monroe was exposed to in Vietnam may trigger the beginnings of chronic insomnia. And that removing the stressful situation may not alleviate the sleep problem. This is an aspect of post-traumatic stress syndrome which I believe needs more careful scrutiny. We tend to blame the problems of Vietnam veterans on their experience of the horrors of war, but the reality may be closer to home.

Once a pattern of disturbed sleep is established, it becomes a kind of self-fulfilling prophecy. Subjects who can't sleep quickly become discouraged and lose confidence in their ability to sleep well, just as they develop anxieties about falling asleep or resuming sleep once they have been awakened. Their anxiety is often aggravated by resorting to impulsive use of alcohol or narcotics (drug use is a persistent problem for many veterans), and by dependency on over-the-counter or prescribed sleep medications.

The veterans I've treated with post-traumatic stress syndrome were all subjected to severe sleep deprivation over a period of time during their stay in the military. By contrast, servicemen and women who flew air missions and were able to return to base each night, showed significantly fewer symptoms. Ground troops, on the other hand, who were isolated on the field of battle and subjected to round-the-clock warfare, carried that stress over day after day. This emotional roller coaster also made them more prone to abusing drugs and alcohol as a way to cope with their stress, further disrupting their sleep cycles.

Fortunately, Monroe's story, like Carla's, has a happy ending. Plus, it provided a fascinating glimpse into one of the least understood aspects of sleep research.

Once I placed Monroe on the nutritional program I developed, bolstered by some basic sleep hygiene, he continued to dream about his wartime experiences. Only now, he reported a feeling of being removed from direct emotional involvement with these nightmarish situations. His sub-conscious began to deal with and eliminate the horrors he had witnessed through his dreams (more on this in later chapters). Gradually, he was beginning to experience less stress, anxiety and depression during the day. After about three to six months of therapy, Monroe's dreams shifted focus and the nightly reliving of his Vietnam experiences started to recede.

Then something very interesting began to occur. Monroe had previously confessed to experiencing a troubling decline in his interest in sex over the years. But after undergoing some months of sleep enhancement therapy, he suddenly began having dreams that were decidedly erotic. Soon, his newly reawakened sexuality wasn't just confined to sleep, and his marriage has since improved dramatically.

Less than a year after we began working together, Monroe was visibly free of the symptoms of post-traumatic stress syndrome, and I'll never forget what he told me. "I feel, for the first time since Vietnam," he said, "that I finally have come home."

It didn't really surprise me that Monroe had been having problems of a sexual nature, and that these problems began to clear when he began to sleep and dream properly. The number one sexual problem is desire disorder, when one person wants sex and the other doesn't. Couples who are on the fast track and aren't sleeping well, often find that intimacy is the first thing to go.

I first met Linda and Charles after my appearance on the Geraldo Show where I had talked about my video, "Eat, Sleep and Be Sexy", Envision, 1989. Linda and Charles had been married for approximately six years. They told me that they had committed themselves in no uncertain terms to a solid and lasting relationship. Their courtship had been perfect, long walks in the park, romantic dinners for two, hours spent gazing into each others eyes. They had many interests and goals they shared, a loving home of their own, someday a house full of children, travel and in the early days sex had been wonderful for them both. In those days, Linda and Charles never imagined their marriage would ever grow stale or be anything less than perfect.

But a year or two into the union, Linda began to realize she had lost her enthusiasm for the sex. This, coincidently, was around the time of the birth of their twins, Kevin & Kyle. It wasn't long after, that Charles also began to notice that something was wrong in the bedroom. Although Charles, too, was somewhat less interested than he had been in the early years of their relationship, he felt if he pursued Linda more aggressively they could recapture the old spark they had once felt for each other. It seemed to Charles that Linda just didn't have any time left for him. He missed the closeness they had shared in the early years. Their marriage had now become less of a storybook romance and more like a prison sentence. Neither was willing to admit there was a problem.

As Linda looked back she thought, perhaps, this had all begun after an argument they had had over money. As for most young couples, finances can often cause disagreements. Linda felt Charles had yelled at her inappropriately when she had nagged him about an unpaid bill. Charles felt guilty after the incident, and told me he had resolved not to lose his temper in the future. For a while, things went well. Each tried to stay calm and be civil, but the physical side of their relationship continued to lack luster.

Charles had been working a lot of overtime in an attempt to improve their financial situation, and Linda decided to work full-time to help out as well, even though she hated leaving the twins in day care. Each told me they were not particularly concerned when their sex life was not intense as it had been. They felt that if the physical side of their marriage lacked the passion it once had, maybe that was to be expected in a marriage. Where once there had been a sensation of being swept away by the moment, now there was only the feeling of monotony. Slowly, Linda began to say no, more frequently, and Charles began to be more insistent.

Linda and Charles began to feel that any expression of affection between them had pretty much ceased to exist. Each confided in me that they began to feel that the romance and mutual affection that had fueled their sex life had ended. As Linda told me, "I'm just too tired at the end of 15 hours of straight work to think about sex."

And small wonder. After I met with Linda and Charles and looked at the kind of schedule that they were each keeping, the problem became clear to me. Each was working outside the home for a minimum of 60 hours per week. Both brought home work at night. It seemed that the amount of time they actually spent together was dwindling almost by the day. Not to mention, that each of them was sleeping less than six hours per night. After a careful evaluation of their lifestyle and development of a program to both enhance sleep and intimacy, Linda and Charles began to experience a warm sensual relationship again. "It's as though we're newlyweds again", Charles confided in me recently.

Carla, Monroe, Linda and Charles each provide insights into aspects of chronic sleep deprivation which manifest themselves in ways that many of us would probably prefer to ignore. What, after all, does our disturbed sleep have in common with that of people who are imprisoned or victims of wars? More than you might imagine. After all, there are certainly other forms of traumatic stress that can disrupt our sleep patterns and cause incredible stresses. For instance, after the San Francisco earthquake a few years ago, many people in the Bay Area found it very difficult to sleep. Aftershocks continued to awaken all of us throughout the night for several weeks. Because of these aftershocks, people were constantly on alert. For many people, they suffered depression, irritability and rage for months after the event. Survivors of automobile accidents, death of a close family member or friend and natural or man-made disasters also show classic symptoms of chronic sleep deprivation.

Not to mention the sudden increase in mass murders. Recent evidence has shown that when levels of serotonin (a critical brain chemical for normal sleep) were measured in normal people, people who had murdered once impulsively, and those who had mass murdered, the mass murderers had significantly lower levels than did those who had murdered only once. Those who had murdered only once had lower levels than did their normal counterparts. This, coupled with the fact that there is a growing body of evidence that links childhood bedwetting, firestarting and animal abuse to mass murders in later years, makes the connection all too clear. We cannot ignore the fact that some people in our society may be chemically predisposed to suffer more severe forms of sleep deprivation. And if these symptoms go unchecked, the sick behavior we are seeing from these mass murderers is the result. We, of course, cannot underestimate the role that the environment plays. However, people who are deprived of a good night's sleep are also extremely suggestible. Perhaps, this, too, impacts homicides, crime, drug and alcohol abuse we are seeing currently in our society. Not surprisingly, sleep deprivation has a long and chilling history as a brainwashing technique, and it is the key ingredient in anyone's attitude— sleep matters!

5   *Bitter Pills*

Just Say "NO!"

Z Z Z Z Z Z Z Z Z Z Z Z Z Z Z Z Z Z Z Z Z Z Z Z Z

As a nation, Americans today consume patented medications to put them to sleep in staggering numbers. Every year, U.S. physicians and psychiatrists write out an estimated 80 million prescriptions for tranquillizers. Indeed, prescription and over-the-counter medications for sleep problems are the most widely sold drugs on the market. Now factor in the sales of medications designed to speed up metabolism and keep you awake, and you can see that sleep loss and its harmful effects constitute our biggest public health problem.

It is now becoming obvious that anyone who takes medications for sleep disorders, stress, weight loss or depression, either over-the-counter or by prescription, is likely to experience a disruption in their sleep cycle. Even antihistamines can disrupt the normal sleep/wake cycle. For example, there are any number of weight-loss products that are known to have amphetamine-like effects. These formulations speed up metabolism as a method of reducing weight. The down side is, under the influence of these drugs, the user may either be unable to successfully fall asleep or is unable to remain in the beneficial stages of sleep for long.

It seems obvious that various forms of "speed" in medications can interfere with sleep patterns, although most people probably don't think of the effects of over-the-counter weight loss formulas in terms of sleep deprivation. Experts even have a term, "medical insomnia", to refer to the effects of certain drugs such as allergy or asthma pills and some forms of nose drops which are known to inhibit sleep.

Earlier in this book, I criticized the use of central nervous system stimulants for children who are prone to hyperactive behavior or learning, discipline or attention problems. While it's true that this potent form of medication can have a calming effect on some children, it strikes me that this is a very destructive approach to the problem.

Some pediatricians don't understand there are very good reasons why many of these children exhibit aggressive or disruptive behavior. These reasons are well documented. We know that food additives, for example, have very marked effects on sensitive children, but child experts have tended to downplay or dismiss these factors in modulating negative behavior. I would like to see more attention paid to the role of artificial sweeteners, for instance, which are present in many processed foods.

Unfortunately, there isn't always support for weaning children away from foods to which they may be allergic. Therefore, the idea that there are simpler, more natural ways of dealing with these problems is still highly unpopular in professional circles.

Anyone who has ever taken antihistamines for a cold or hay fever knows that these drugs can make you extremely sleepy, which is why their manufacturers use them as a basis for sleep products. Not surprisingly, sleeping medications sold in pharmacies and supermarkets without prescription generally contain an antihistamine.

Here, I want to repeat my assertion that all sleep is not necessarily equal. And drugged sleep is far inferior to natural sleep. Obviously, anyone who is taking some form of stimulant or antihistamine can expect these substances to significantly interfere with their natural sleep patterns. What is perhaps less well known, tranquilizers and sleeping pills can also have harmful side effects that negatively affect the body's ability to induce normal sleep.

Most of these drugs (and I should include alcohol, tobacco, caffeine and even artificial sweeteners in the list) tend to negatively affect the natural sleep cycle. They have the net result of driving the body artificially into the deeper stages of sleep and, consequently, depriving the sleeper of valuable REM sleep.

In other words, while sedatives may make it easier for you to fall asleep, the kind of sleep that you experience is not necessarily restorative. If you don't get both the proper <u>quantity</u> of sleep and the right <u>quality</u> of sleep, you won't awaken feeling rested and refreshed. Likewise, people who use sedatives, sleeping medications, alcohol or excessive amounts of caffeine, frequently complain about this problem. Such individuals commonly awaken feeling "hung over". And, if you aren't waking up in the morning feeling rested, rejuvenated and ready to tackle a new day, you probably aren't getting enough proper sleep.

Irritability and depression also occur frequently when our sleep cycle is interrupted, leading to another vicious circle. In recent times, many women who suffered from premenstrual syndrome have been given tranquilizers for these symptoms. The prevailing attitude of the medical community for many years was, if a woman continued to complain about her symptoms, more tranquilizers were in order. Failing that, doctors resorted to more radical measures, hysterectomies. While we've seen some improvement in doctors' attitudes to such symptoms fairly recently, I think it's safe to say that this sort of backward thinking still persists today in some medical circles.

People who have to rouse themselves from sleep after a night spent under the influence of these and similar medications often complain of feeling even more fatigued, depressed and irritable than they were when they went to bed. However, they often don't connect the use of these medications with their feelings. They may think that they are depressed and irritable because of a particular life situation. Then they are concerned that they won't be able to sleep, or they might overeat. So they turn to their trusted medications, and the vicious circle repeats itself. Perhaps, I should call it a vicious spiral, because this pattern will only perpetuate the same downward trend.

While there are relatively few scientific studies on the side effects of tranquilizers and sleep medications prescribed for sleep, in recent years there has been a wave of public unrest concerning the potential harm of these drugs. Consumers, in increasing numbers, are finally beginning to connect their negative experiences when taking these medications with the medications themselves. This emerging trend, to pay more attention to what our bodies are telling us about the use of these medications, is one in which I am, frankly, delighted. It is my personal belief that not a single one of these medications have any place in long-term treatment for any person. And, in fact, most of these medications were designed for short-term use only. Unfortunately, some physicians have continued to prescribe them month after month, even though the evidence suggests that they are not effective after a short period of time.

Although the pharmaceutical industry has been understandably reluctant to fund studies about the clinical aspects of this national problem, I think it's fairly obvious that many of the behavioral aberrations tied to the abuse of these drugs betray many of the familiar symptoms of sleep deprivation. If you have any doubts about this, I suggest you refer to a copy of the Physician's Desk Reference (PDR) and its list of side effects associated with any number of sleeping medications or tranquilizers. You may be shocked to discover symptoms you perhaps have experienced for yourself which are widely published in the medical record.

Side effects, of course, are just one aspect of the problem. Taking these drugs can be fatal, either from overdose, accidents caused while under their influence, suicide or even murder. Nevertheless, these products remain on the shelves and are widely prescribed by many doctors.

While the negative effects associated with some of the older tranquilizers are fairly well known (thanks largely to best sellers and television movies on the subject, rather than any response from the medical community at large), others have still not come under the kind of scrutiny they deserve. The trouble is none of the tranquilizers and sleeping medications come without side effects, and the side effects, as you can see, may be devastating.

Worse than taking these drugs is trying to get off them. Detoxification from long-term use of sleeping pills or tranquilizers is proven to be extremely difficult. WARNING: DO NOT STOP TAKING ANY MEDICATION WITHOUT A DOCTOR'S SUPERVISION. Some experts even maintain that these products are harder to withdraw from than notorious "street" drugs, such as, heroin and "crack" cocaine. I would venture to say that there are more people addicted to prescription drugs than to so-called recreational or street drugs. We are telling our children to "just say no". Perhaps, it's time someone considered taking this campaign to the pharmaceutical companies.

Some of the side effects of these pharmaceutical drugs may even be fatal, either to the persons taking the drugs or to other people who happen to be around them. Any number of lawsuits have been filed in recent years by surviving relatives of murder victims with the contention that the killer was taking some prescription drug. These are difficult cases to prove, since the subjects were usually depressed or violent before they started taking the drugs. But the sheer volume of litigation on this issue would indicate that for some people, at least, many of the most popular (and, need I add, lucrative) drugs can have a drastic impact on behavior.

Proponents of pharmaceutical sleep aids argue that sleeping medications which don't cause aftereffects or drowsiness, don't interact dangerously with alcohol and other drugs, can't possibly be harmful. But there is plenty of evidence that virtually all pharmaceutical sleep medications have these effects on at least some of the people who take them.

The elderly, who take a large portion of these medications, are at particular risk because their systems do not metabolize drugs as readily as younger people. When a partial amount of the drug is left in a person's system, it is known as the "half-life" of the drug. If this excretion time is lengthened, as is the case in many elderly, the half-life is also lengthened, leading to a dangerous build-up of the drug. This, in combination with other prescription medication, can spell disaster for those concerned. If proof were needed, there have been a number of cases where elderly patients were taken off medication with a remarkable improvement in memory and mood.

Let me state that I am not making a blanket denunciation of pharmaceutical companies, physicians or drugs. I do, however, think that it is only ethical and prudent for physicians and pharmaceutical companies to put the welfare of the patient ahead of their profits.

Antidepressant medications, that increase serotonin levels are now widely used in the treatment of depression. Although I recommend prudence in the use of any antidepressant, it has been my experience that, when properly prescribed by a knowledgeable physician, these drugs can be quite remarkable. It is certainly not appropriate for everyone, but it can be effective, particularly those that increase serotonin levels. At the same time, many of these medications seem to have negative effects in some cases. One of the side effects seems to be a feeling of agitation. Generally, when serotonin levels are increased, people will experience what is known as REM rebound, an increase in the dreaming state of sleep. This can often leave the sleeper with the feeling that he was awake all night. His brain is literally "zooming" out of control. In my experience, this generally lasts about a week. Interestingly enough, although the sleeper may feel he hasn't slept a wink, he often reports feeling more awake and alert during the day. Another problem may be the result of overzealous physicians who prescribe antidepressant medications incorrectly.

Finally, if you're concerned about your intake of sleep medication, it may help you to know that researchers have proven many people, given one sleeping pill or another, fall asleep before the medication has had a chance to have any physiological effect. In other words, sleeping pills function as a sort of placebo for many people who take them, and so, constitute not just an unnecessary expense, but also an unwarranted robbing of precious sleep reserves. AGAIN, DO NOT STOP ANY MEDICATION WITHOUT FIRST CONSULTING YOUR DOCTOR. IT IS CRITICAL THAT YOUR DOCTOR MONITOR YOU WHILE TAPERING OFF OF ANY OF THESE DRUGS.

All in all, the prospect of a tranquilizer's and sleeping pill's potential for harm is a grim one. On the other hand, there is one natural sedative which has proven to be highly beneficial, as I can vouch from my own personal experience. It is the amino acid, L-tryptophan. (See Appendix B.)

Most people can learn to enjoy the benefits of natural, restorative sleep without the use of either sleeping pills or tranquilizers. In later chapters I will discuss ways to have a restful, refreshing sleep—sleep matters!

6 *Dreamscape*

The Nightly Timetable of Sleep

Z Z Z Z Z Z Z Z Z Z Z Z Z Z Z Z Z Z Z Z Z Z Z Z

No one seems to know precisely why we sleep, or for that matter, why we sleep the way we do. Considering that we spend approximately one third of our lives engaged in slumber, you would think we would know more about the function of sleep. Why do we need it so much, and why can't we get by with less of it.

We do know, however, that sleep helps repair the daily wear and tear on consciousness, helps us to assimilate all the information we soak up each day and facilitates the storage of memory. While it is true, as one prominent researcher has pointed out, that "the only known function of sleep is to promote wakefulness the next day", what that "wakefulness" implies is not so well understood.

But one thing we all do know is that we feel at our best when we get a good night's sleep. Of course, some people seem to require more sleep, and others appear to be able to get by with less. But most of us would agree that going without sleep for an indefinite period of time is a prescription for disaster. This much is sure: sleep is good for us, and the right kind of sleep is good for us in very important ways. However self-evident, it's a fact that sleep constitutes a profoundly restorative process, and a growing body of research supports the view that we ignore the benefits of a good night's sleep at our own peril. And, when I refer to a good night's sleep, I am describing the quality, as well as the quantity, of sleep you get. In order to wake up, both mentally and physically refreshed, both are essential.

Let's look first at the nightly schedule or timetable, if you will, of normal sleep. Prior to falling asleep, we experience what may be the most mysterious of sleep processes, technically known as the "hypnagogic" stage (that is, "inducing or leading to sleep"). How this brief interval of being half-awake and half-asleep can be useful in determining the quality of your sleep will be explained in later chapters.

What happens after the hypnogogic state was pretty much a closed book until about 40 years ago. The mystery of sleep began to unfold in the 1950's when researchers discovered a startling discontinuity in sleep rhythms. Scientists at the University of Chicago and Stanford University identified two major, differentiated, physiological processes that occur during the sleep cycle. They found that at certain times during the night, the sleep subjects they tested began to experience what was eventually termed "rapid eye movement" (REM) sleep. The majority of the sleep cycle was spent in what is now known as "non-rapid eye movement" (non-REM) sleep.

When we sleep, we fluctuate back and forth from REM to non-REM sleep throughout the night, in a tightly choreographed rhythm of sleep patterns. (See Diagrams 1 and 2). Non-REM sleep, which takes up about three-quarters of total sleeping time, comes first and is termed "quiescent", still or inactive. Blood pressure and body temperature drop, the heart rate and metabolism slow, and muscles relax.

Diagram 1

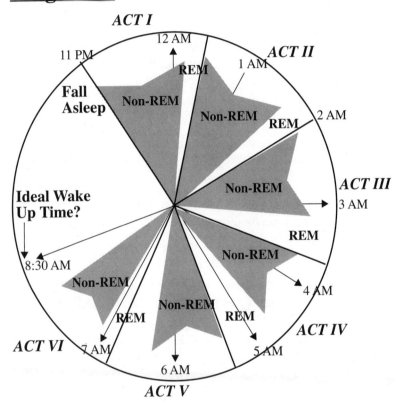

A Night's Sleep in Six Acts

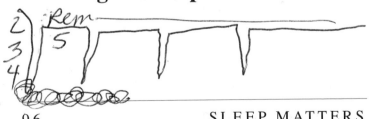

SLEEP MATTERS

Diagram 2

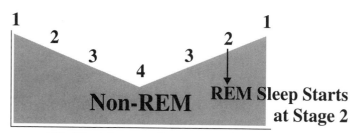

70-90 minute sleep cycle

Next, we enter the first of a series of five distinct and recurring stages of sleep. Stages One through Four consist of non-REM sleep, while Stage Five consists of REM sleep. This fifth phase is the stage during which we dream. As a rule, a person passes through all five stages of sleep approximately every 70 to 90 minutes during the night, repeating the cycle roughly six or seven times on the average.

<u>Stage One</u> - a light, drifting sleep - accounts for about five percent of the entire night's tally, and usually lasts from one to seven minutes per occurrence. <u>Stage Two</u> - somewhat deeper sleep - makes up the greatest amount of time, about 45 to 55 percent. <u>Stage Three</u> - another five percent or so of sleep time - takes us even deeper into

sleep. The deepest, "dead-to-the-world" sleep occurs in <u>Stage Four</u>. Here, an interesting thing happens. The sleeper begins to drift upward into Stage Three sleep, and then to Stage Two sleep, just before entering that all-important dream phase known as REM sleep. (See diagrams 1 & 2).

REM activity takes up the remaining 20 to 25 percent of the sleep schedule. In some ways, REM sleep is much like wakefulness with at least one crucial difference. Our muscles twitch, our eyes move rapidly behind closed lids, our blood pressure rises and falls, and our heartbeat speeds up and slows down. But our bodies remain rigid until we reenter non-REM sleep. So, although, we may dream of physical activity, we are altogether unable to act out what we dream.

After each period of REM sleep, the sleeper reenters non-REM sleep—first Stage Two, then Three, then Four, and then back up to Stage Three, to Stage Two—then proceeds back into the dream period of Stage Five. This process is repeated over and over again during the night. The brain returns to dreaming approximately five times during the night. The number of these dream periods being roughly determined by the length of time we spend asleep.

As the nighttime hours go by, the percentage of REM time in each 70-90 minute "act" of sleep continues to lengthen (see diagram 1). That's partly why most of us seem to remember more of our dreams from the early morning hours. Ultimately, the percentage of time during the last sleep period that is spent in REM sleep is much greater than it was in the first phase of sleep. A sleeper may eventually spend as much as 20 minutes at a time in the dreaming stage of sleep.

Over the years since the discovery of REM and non-REM sleep patterns, researchers have untangled a web of interrelated functions in these two complementary sleep processes. Non-REM sleep appears to be very important for ensuring our physical well-being, while REM sleep appears to influence our mental health. Put another way, non-REM has a physiological function, and REM sleep has a psychological function. If, as one expert suggests, "the body needs rest, but the brain needs sleep", then REM sleep emerges as a critical factor in the quality of sleep we get.

Sleep, in general, has been described as a sort of overnight "battery charge" for the body. Both bone formation and physical growth accelerate during sleep, while cell rejuvenation continues pretty much uninterrupted 24 hours a day. Therefore, it is speculated that sleep is not, strictly speaking, biologically necessary. Rather, it seems to have originated as a survival tactic during the early stages of animal evolution when the mental processes of learning perception were perfected during sleep.

Some experts believe that REM sleep operates like a safety valve. It provides a way for the brain to process events from the previous day which are emotionally charged and which we don't have the time or energy to deal with while we are awake. Researchers have come to view this function of REM sleep as a form of "mental housekeeping". Studies show that processing emotions and memories through dreaming may be vital to psychological well-being. It is also known that subjects deprived of REM sleep will spend more time in that state during the following night. It's as though the body intuitively understands that this particular period of sleep is a critical factor in mental health.

In recent years, some sleep specialists have even come to the conclusion that there is a particular structure to sleep that allows us, through our dreams, to cope with the stresses of everyday life and possibly determine our future actions. Studies have suggested that, in fact, dream material is presented in a decidedly fixed order. As we sleep, our brains repeatedly return to processing the previous day's information, each time putting it together in new ways.

During the first dream of the night, the mind presents us with an overview of the problems it wishes to solve. The second and third dream states then begin to integrate our current situation with similar experiences from the past. These experiences are then reconciled with underlying emotions connected to both present and past events. The fourth dream stage is concerned with decision-making about problems and events we may face in the future. The fifth and final dream stage then consolidates all the information from the previous four stages and presents us with a solution of sorts, often in symbolic form.

In a sense, dreams offer a premonition of impending anxieties and give us the skills necessary to handle them. In my opinion, it would be virtually impossible to cope with the many stresses of every day life without REM periods of sleep. And if dreaming is a means of solving the many problems we face each day, then it comes as no surprise that most dreams will center around stressful events, and that relatively few dreams are concerned with success or good fortune, unless, of course, the dreamer finds these situations stressful.

Many dream experts believe that the emotions we express through our dreams help prepare us for future ordeals, from final exams to job interviews and business presentations. Just about everyone has nightmares related to achievement and performance. My own experience certainly bears this out. For example, I vividly recall a dream I had the night before I was to speak before a number of my colleagues at an important medical conference. In my dream "rehearsal", when I began to speak at the podium in front of me, it tumbled to the floor. As I continued, no one could hear me, people began to get up and leave, and my lecture was a shambles. But when I actually spoke at the conference the next day, I was braced for any such possibility, and none of the disasters I'd anticipated occurred. As a matter of fact, the audience was extremely receptive. Perhaps, because of my "dream rehearsal".

Other studies have confirmed that people who are about to face a traumatic life event spend more time in REM sleep, but not always to the same effect. In one sleep laboratory, volunteers who were subjected to an ego-threatening experience prior to sleep and who then spent time dreaming about the experience, were found to be less tense on waking than those who did not dream after a similar experience.

It appears that even the most fundamental life events are rehearsed in dreams. One study of pregnant women showed that subjects who dreamed of problems connected with being pregnant and the birth of a child, in fact, experienced easier and briefer labor and deliveries.

There is a large body of evidence that suggests dreams provide a psychological release during which the right hemisphere of the brain deals with suppressed feelings of anxiety, rage and hostility. So, if we are facing serious challenges, like, say, cramming for an exam, our brains compensate by increasing the amount of REM sleep. On the other hand, when subjects are deprived of REM sleep, learning ability declines, and they are less capable of coping with emotional problems.

When REM-deprived individuals are allowed to sleep again, they experience what is known as "REM rebound". In other words, they compensate by increasing the amount of time they subsequently spent in REM sleep. If sleeping subjects are repeatedly awakened prior to entering a period of REM sleep, when allowed to sleep again, they will travel much more quickly than usual through the first four stages of sleep to catch up on REM sleep.

There also have been numerous studies which showed that when animals and humans are deprived of REM sleep they grow more anxious, irritable, and restless. In other words, there is an alteration in our attitude. It's no wonder that so many people these days are showing signs of psychological wear and tear.

Researchers have also shown that REM sleep is critical in the learning process. REM sleep is not only needed to help us assimilate the stressful events of a day, it is also a key factor in cognition. Researchers found that when sleep subjects were shown a series of every day objects and asked to memorize them, those who spent the greatest amount of time dreaming had the best memory recall. When you appreciate just how important REM sleep is to learning and to mental health, it's enough to make you wonder if the poor classroom performance of so many school children these days may not be rooted in deprivation of REM sleep. Perhaps we should consider starting school a bit later in the mornings to allow our children one more period of REM.

So, we've looked at what constitutes normal sleep, but now we need to know more about what happens when we don't get enough of it. Scientists place sleep deprivation in various categories. With total sleep deprivation, subjects are deprived of any sleep at all for periods of from 60 to even 200 hours (that's more than a week). With partial sleep deprivation, subjects are deprived of REM sleep over a period of several nights which, in fact, is what most Americans may experience over a period of *years*.

Total deprivation of both non-REM and REM sleep can cause any or all of the following symptoms: fatigue, irritability, decreased concentration, inaccurate perception, disorientation, deterioration of motor-task performance, depression and hallucinations. In certain predisposed individuals, it may provoke psychotic episodes accompanied by bouts of screaming, sobbing, incoherent speech, delusions and paranoia. In my opinion, this is a pretty fair description of how most commuters behave in the middle of rush hour traffic.

It's a safe bet that most of us who have suffered some form of sleep deprivation are familiar with the symptoms. At such moments, we may experience events as though they are happening to someone else, at a great distance or as if occurring underwater. This sense of disorientation is also a symptom of jet lag, the feeling that you aren't exactly where you should be, though you know logically that you are.

The impression that what was once familiar has somehow become unreal is probably caused by subtle or not-so-subtle changes in your sleep schedule which, in turn, alter your interior body clock. This circadian rhythm, as it is called, dictates when you wake and when you sleep, and it is controlled by a tiny organ in the brain known as the pineal gland. The internal body clock can be set back one hour earlier or two hours later without causing too much disorientation, but when the time difference is more like five to eight hours the results for weary travellers can be psychologically devastating. Left to itself, readjustment of the body clock can take several weeks to accomplish. Meanwhile, the body is registering the all-too-familiar symptoms of sleep deprivation.

It's a measure of our lack of understanding where sleep is concerned that only in recent years have psychiatric studies pinpointed the real causes of holiday depression, also known as the "winter blues". It usually begins soon after the Christmas holidays, and it is especially prevalent in climates where long months of gray and overcast weather are the rule. For people who suffer the symptoms of what is now known as Seasonal Affective Disorder (SAD), this syndrome can have such a devastating effect that many of those afflicted have to retreat from work and social activity for as long as four or five months at a stretch.

Because our sleep cycle is in part controlled by our perception of light and dark, brain chemicals can be altered in winter months. Some individuals seem predisposed to depression during the winter months. Those suffering from SAD have been successfully treated with light therapy. This treatment, in affect, resets their internal clock, and it nudges those afflicted into an early spring.

While the symptoms of SAD may seem extreme, many of us in more southern climates are probably suffering the same effects to a lesser degree. I am convinced that in too many homes, the contrast between light and darkness is simply not sharp enough. Street lights, headlights or the glow from the television you fall asleep in front of can all play a part in blurring the distinction between waking and sleep. In addition, many people work indoors for most of the day, exposed to inadequate artificial light, rather than natural light.

It is now known that when transitions from light to dark are not sufficiently extreme, the production of key brain chemicals associated with the transition to sleep are affected. So once again, the invention of the light bulb has not only decreased the hours of sleep most of us get, but has also decreased the contrast from light to dark that is so crucial to normal brain function and normal sleep. It has tampered with our sleep patterns and circadian rhythms and interfered with our ability to dream.

The good news here is that we can undue the damage of insufficient sleep. On the first night of restored sleep, someone who is sleep-deprived will begin by dropping quickly down to Stage

Four sleep, at the expense of time spent in stages One, Two, and Three. The body, in other words, can't wait to get to the much needed deeper stages of sleep. Then it is periodically interrupted with periods of REM sleep.

On the second night of restored sleep following a period of sleep deprivation, Stage Five, REM sleep rebounds with the result that REM sleep exceeds the amount the subject was experiencing prior to sleep deprivation.

This period of catching up on REM sleep usually lasts for two to four days, at which time the subject begins feeling progressively better. This might explain the use of sleep deprivation as a treatment for depression. Sure enough, when depressed individuals are deprived of sleep for a very limited time, they begin by experiencing a period of normal REM sleep, leaving them less depressed. What, in fact, may be happening is that their depression is alleviated because of their enhanced abilities for problem-solving while in REM sleep.

Partial, but chronic, sleep deprivation can have many insidious and dangerous effects, in my opinion. People who are prevented from having adequate REM sleep night after night, either because they are not getting enough sleep or because they are ingesting medications or food additives which interfere with REM sleep, are at the greatest risk. Both children and adults who are thus sleep deprived can become hyperactive, emotionally unstable, vulnerable to mood swings and quick to overreact. In this state, many people will "act out" when confronted with trivial irritations which merely serve as a surrogate target for their unexpressed rage. If this hostility is not expressed, they may internalize their feelings and become more severely depressed.

Partial sleep deprivation has also been correlated with overactivity, excessive appetite and exaggerated sexual behavior in studies of REM-deprived animals. This may go a long way to explain why couples who find themselves operating according to different sleep schedules often fight about sex. As I mentioned earlier, "desire disorder", as it's fashionably known, is the primary complaint in most relationships. In doing the research for the *Eat, Sleep and Be Sexy* video, we found that sleep deprivation was a major factor in sexual desire. By correcting this sleep imbalance with proper diet, sexual desire returned to normal in almost all cases.

While all of this discussion about REM and non-REM sleep is important to understanding what constitutes good sleep, that still doesn't mean we've licked the problem. Ultimately, the solution to sleep deprivation lies in the complex, metabolic chemistry of sleep. (See Appendix C).

Normal, restorative sleep is the key ingredient to a balanced, happy life—sleep matters!

SLEEP TIPS

- Be consistent about your sleep schedule, try not to vary your bedtime more than one hour early or two hours late.

- Develop regular habits and stick to them.

- Sleep 8-10 hours per night, experiment until you find out what feels best for you.

- Increase your sleep time during periods of increased stress.

- Sleep in a dark, quiet and cool room.

- Invest in a good mattress and bedding to insure the best sleep possible.

- Make sleep a high priority in your life.

- Discuss the importance of sleep with your family and friends, share your new found knowledge.

- Minimize sleep interruptions whenever possible.

- Take naps if you are unable to get your normal amount of sleep.

- Consider sleep as the most important factor in your mental well-being.

- Eat a well balanced diet (more about this in later chapters).

- Exercise in the afternoon whenever possible (more about this in later chapters).

- Unwind prior to falling asleep such as reading or watching television, something that you find relaxing.

- Take a hot bath and allow time to cool down before falling asleep, this cooling down signals the body it is time to fall asleep.

- Find some form of regular stress reduction and stick with it.

- Give yourself a little quiet time before going to bed, time to relax and unwind, you deserve it.

- Establish a sleep routine—do things in the same order, this helps signal the brain it is nearly time to fall asleep (this is especially important with children).

- Use a sleep mask to help establish a distinction between light and dark.

- When you awaken in the morning, turn on lights and open drapes, even spend a few minutes outside in the natural light. This will help to reset the bodyclock for the next night's sleep.

- When you arise, wash your face or shower to help you wake up (it takes a few minutes to completely awaken).
- Avoid large meals of protein late at night.
- Talk to your doctor about eliminating tranquilizers and sleeping medications.
- Don't exercise right before bedtime.
- Practice moderation in your consumption of alcohol and caffeine—completely avoid all artificial sweeteners.
- If you smoke, talk to your doctor about new ways to quit.
- Have a good night's sleep, you deserve it and remember—sleep matters!

7 *Uptight, All Night*

Too Stressed to Sleep

ZZZZZZZZZZZZZZZZZZZZZZZZZZ

The average American is working
between 30 and 80 hours outside the home per
week. He or she commutes to and from work,
then returns home to deal with housework, cook-
ing, dishes, children and an endless supply of
homework that always seems to require a parent's help. Add to this, the stress of living in an
economy none of us seem to be able to afford,
and you have the American dream. Or has it
become the American nightmare?

The typical day begins something like this. The
alarm rings at 5:30 a.m., you roll over, yawn and
press snooze thinking, "Please let me have just a
few more minutes of sleep." Nine minutes later,
you hear the sound you've grown to hate.

Exhausted, you roll out of bed thinking, "I've got to start getting more sleep." You promise yourself you're going to sleep in on the weekend. You stagger into the shower, get dressed and start breakfast. Other family members have also started to get up. Everyone looks tired and acts cranky. The kids don't want to get up for school. No one is in a good mood. Someone, usually the wife, makes lunches, and everyone leaves for their commute to work or school.

The day passes much like most. You feel stressed and exhausted. But you compensate for this stress and fatigue by drinking coffee, diet sodas or overeating. Somehow, it ends, and you return home after fighting the traffic, to find a houseful of chores that all require your attention. The laundry needs doing, dinner needs to be cooked, children are grumpy and fighting with each other. You wonder, "Why can't everyone just cooperate?" By the time everyone is fed and in bed, it's 11:00 p.m., and there are still dishes to do and another two loads of laundry. Not to mention, you still have those reports that have to be finished for your boss tomorrow. Finally, about 12:30 a.m., you fall into bed for your well deserved five hours of sleep. You don't really have much time to talk with your spouse about anything but the chores and bills, much less, think about having sex.

After what seems like an endless period of time, it's finally Friday night. It's no wonder TGIF has become our National prayer. Perhaps, you stay up just a little later tonight, after all you can always sleep in and catch up over the weekend. Saturday morning rolls around, and you do sleep in until about 9:00 or 10:00 a.m. if you are lucky. You feel a little better. You still have all the chores that have gone undone all week, like the yard work, washing the cars, taking yourself and the kids in for haircuts, clothes shopping and the like. The day seems to fly by, and before you know it, you're in front of the TV with movies for the evening. You stay up a little later tonight because your body is on a 25-hour clock rather than a 24- hour clock, and you think, "I still have Sunday to sleep in." You awaken Sunday morning late, and either relax at home or get dressed and go to church. Your day is filled with more chores, and you fall into bed Sunday night unable to fall asleep quickly. You awaken even more exhausted on Monday morning to start all over again.

As I pointed out in earlier chapters, I believe that sleep deprivation and the stress that goes with it are of critical importance for most people today. It is the number one problem facing Americans today. Lack of sleep is affecting every aspect of our lives. From children who are having learning difficulties to teens who are using drugs and alcohol. It can cause PMS in women and physical abusiveness in men. It is making us a nation of moody, irritable and often, confused people. It is sapping our creativity, as well as, increasing criminal behavior. And it is devastating to our economy, as well as, to industry. We all have too much to do, and few of us are getting enough rest. This spells **stress** with a capital **S**!

We all experience stress at one time or another. Essentially, there are two kinds of stress. There is good stress, and there is bad stress. When an athlete is preparing for an olympic event, he, for the most part, is experiencing good stress. That is, the stress he chooses to help him compete in a more aggressive way. Primarily, the athlete imposes physical stress on his body because he has learned that this form of stress will culminate in a better trained body. Thus, the swimmer swims miles in an effort to increase his or her time and endurance. The weight trainer continues to lift heavier and heavier weights in an effort to continually increase his strength, and so forth. This is a form of self-imposed stress that he or she uses to their advantage. However, if the athlete is being stressed by outside influences, such as an overzealous parent, this can quickly become a bad form of stress. There are also other forms of "bad" stress, such as, stresses caused by our environment. This may cause stress on our body from say a poor diet or air quality. Financial stresses also fall into the category of bad stresses.

Often, it is difficult to tell the difference between good and bad stress. As I stated earlier, an athlete who has trained his body, but is being pressured by an over enthusiastic parent may not have dealt with the emotional stress of competition. This can often lead to disastrous consequences.

Early man was given an instinct for survival known as fight or flight. In other words, if a large lion were confronting him, he would see only two options. Stay and fight the lion if he were cornered, or flee if that option seemed more viable. During this process, his entire metabolic rate would increase. He would secrete massive amounts of adrenaline. His peripheral blood vessels would constrict, thus, elevating his blood pressure and flow of blood to his brain. Other glands would also secrete hormones, and his muscles would mobilize glycogen stores for quick energy needs while fatty-acids would be mobilized for long-term energy needs. Although few of us are faced with lions on a daily basis, in many ways, the same physiological response is occurring. For instance, take the person who is confronted by an angry and unreasonable boss on a daily basis. He may feel like running or fighting. Except, in modern day society, we all know we can't "fight" the boss, and running out of the office is generally frowned upon. Although, I must confess, I have wanted to do both on more than one occasion.

So what happens to our brain chemistry when all this adrenaline is rushing and screaming at us to fight or run? After the influx of massive amounts of adrenaline, energy stores are used, and brain serotonin levels are also depleted. This happens even with small amounts of adrenaline. For instance, if you are driving home in rush hour traffic and people continually cut you off or stop suddenly, almost causing you to have an accident, you will more than likely feel stress. Modern man is faced with almost continuous stress, and he has no ability to either fight or flee. When brain serotonin levels are low, an interruption in the normal sleep cycle is the result. Lack of sleep subsequently causes the individual to be more emotionally fragile, and it decreases the ability of that individual to handle stress effectively. Thus, a vicious downward spiral begins.

We've already talked about physical stress. The athlete who must condition his body continually in order to compete is experiencing physical stress. There are other forms of unexpected stress for which we may not always be prepared. For instance, if we are in a traffic accident and injuries occur, this produces a stress on our physical being. An elderly person who is not in the best physical condition may be attacked by a mugger and forced to run. This would create a form of physical stress. We are bombarded by all sorts of physical stress on a daily basis. Anytime we ask our bodies to do something it is not conditioned to do, this causes physical stress. Anything from exercise to shoveling snow from a driveway to illness can cause physical stress. Occasionally, physical stress can lead to death. If, for instance, the man who was shoveling snow from his driveway was in poor physical condition, and he overexerted, he may cause a heart attack or a stroke, simply by asking his body to perform a rigorous task for which he was not physically prepared.

Physical stress places demands on our bodies for which we must be prepared. It is only logical to assume that the person who has taken the time to condition his/her body will meet the demands placed on it in a more effective way than the person who has not taken the time or energy to prepare his/her body. When physical stress occurs, the body produces adrenaline. The heart must be able to handle this influx of adrenaline, so the individual will be able to either flee or stand and fight.

It is always wise to take notice of a conditioned athlete who has taken the time and energy to plan a program of conditioning which will allow him to better use his body in the event of an emergency. One of the best and most effective ways to fight physical, as well as, emotional stress is a planned program of regular exercise.

*To some degree, all stress is emotional. I know in my own experience that emotional stress can be devastating both emotionally and physically. I believe it can even be life threatening. When L-tryptophan was removed from the market after it's contamination, this lesson began to really hit home for me. I had spent the seven years prior to that time researching, writing and marketing my book, **The Pre-Menstrual Solution, How to Tame the Shrew in You, Arrow Press, 1987**. I had flown back to New York to appear on the Donahue Show in mid-October of 1989, and* *that's when my period of stress began. On the flight home, our troubles started. The plane was overcrowded, and it was full of people who had been stranded for over 24 hours in an airport out of the country. They were tired, irritable and did not speak the language. Add to that the air conditioning problems the plane was having, and the fact that many of the other passengers had not bathed for several days, and I'm sure you can begin to get the picture. As we took off, the plane was shaking so badly that my daughter, Jill, turned to me and said, "I guess if our seats fall through the floor, we'll land in the luggage compartment?" She was reading my mind! We arrived home at 3:00 a.m. in the San Francisco airport, hot and tired. The next day, Jill and I slept in and tried to recover from our jet lag. My husband, Michael, had been working all day, but returned home early. We were just about to prepare dinner and sit down to watch the world series when the entire house began to shake. The Loma Prieta earthquake of 7.1 on the Richter scale had arrived. I can't begin to explain the kind of stress this produced. Aftershocks continued to wake us up from our sleep every few minutes for weeks on end. We had no electrical power, no water, and I had been out-of-town so there wasn't much food in the house. All the neighbors pulled together, and, in some ways, we became much closer. One of our neighbors began to have contractions (she was nine months pregnant), and we began to think the delivery would occur at my house by candlelight. Fortunately, the stork waited another day, and she made it to the hospital. For weeks after this, I feared leaving my house, and I felt almost constant anxiety, as did almost everyone in the San Francisco Bay Area. We were lucky. We had little damage, and all of us were home at the time. But even though all was well with us personally, we continued to feel stressed.*

The aftershocks continued for several weeks, and just as I was beginning to feel somewhat better, I received a telephone call from a reporter in New Mexico. The L-tryptophan nightmare began. I had strongly recommended the use of this powerful amino acid in my first book. People, I was told, were now developing a rare blood disorder called Eosinophilia Myalgia Syndrome as a result of the contamination. (See Appendix B.)

My telephone would not quit ringing. Reporters were calling my house day and night wanting to send crews over to interview me. The press began to have a field day with this problem. Women began to call from all over the country, at all hours of the day and night. I'm not talking about a few women. I'm talking about thousands of calls, each leaving their name and number and expecting to speak with me personally. My telephone bill was astronomical. Everyone expected me to call them back. Most women wanted to continue to take this food supplement as it had dramatically improved their lives. But because the FDA had recalled it, women were unable to obtain it. Many women were truly desperate, and they told me horror stories of having abused children or attempted suicide before using this amino acid successfully. Many women felt they would rather risk dying than go back to living the way they had before taking L-tryptophan. Some men and women were angry, and they suggested that I had lied in my book. Or that somehow, I had known that this would be a problem. Some people filed law suits, even though the first amendment protects against such suits. As it turned out, accord-

ing to the Center for Disease Control, the problems caused by L-tryptophan were a result of a contamination caused by one raw materials manufacturer. However, by the time this was discovered, several months after the original reports in the media, the story was old news, and little was reported about the actual cause. Not only was I receiving thousands of telephone calls from those who had taken L-tryptophan, but I was also hearing from bookstores, the Food and Drug Administration and the media. Then, the financial stress began. I believe that had it not been for the fact that I obtained L-tryptophan for my personal use through the Canadian market, I would not have been able to cope. I know that stress occurs when you feel out of control with a situation. The reality, of course, is that we really have little control over what happens to us, and that we must be physically and mentally prepared to handle life's challenges.

Not all emotional stresses are as devastating as the one I experienced, and some, of course, are much worse. The sum of many small stresses throughout the day can spell disaster for many of us. What is stressful for one person, often causes no stress for another. For instance, talking on national television has never caused me to feel stress. In fact, the reverse is often true. I find the experience exhilarating. My husband, on the other hand, says he would rather swim the Atlantic ocean rather than appear in any way in the media. Even the same activity can cause stress under one set of circumstances and no stress under another. Take, for instance, a doctor who gave a talk in front of a group of nurses, he felt confident and completely in control. Since the nurses were his subordinates, his pulse rate, blood pressure and metabolic rate remained constant. In other words, he was relaxed and perfectly composed, not in the least rattled or on edge.

But when the doctor gave the same speech to a group of his colleagues, his peers, some of whom were physicians with more experience and knowledge, he wasn't nearly so cool or controlled. In this situation, he believed that his competency was on the line. Thus, the same speech produced quite different results in his level of stress. The doctor's pulse quickened, his blood pressure increased and his metabolic rate became elevated. He was under stress.

Thus, we can begin to see how emotional stresses can have a physical impact on the body. Moreover, had the doctor been worried about losing his job, he might have perspired or his throat might have gone dry or even the timbre of his voice might have changed.

There are, of course, other forms of emotional stress that can be devastating. For example, the sudden death of a loved one, a divorce, the loss of a job, the rejection of a friend or loved one, the failure to pass an exam after much study, learning you are about to die from an incurable disease, etc. Any of these kinds of stresses can cause serious emotional and physical damage. If you aren't already ill, you may become ill because of the changes in your sleep cycle which occur as a result of this kind of stress. If you are ill, you may experience an increase in symptoms because loss of sleep negatively affects the immunological system.

One of the most insidious forms of stress and one that plagues our society today is the daily stress we all face, on-the-job deadlines, sleep deprived co-workers, bosses who are irritable and moody, traffic, lines in grocery stores and banks, competition, financial stresses, children and spouses. The bottom line for many people is that we feel we just don't have enough time to accomplish what we want or what is essential. Some of this "chronic stress" just comes with the territory of work, and some people appear to thrive on this kind of environment with no apparent ill effects. However, this kind of stress can be particularly intense for those who are already sleep deprived. Add to the stress of the working world the stress on the home front, and it's easy to see the potential for disaster. The Japanese culture is one of the few cultures on the planet that may actually be more stressed than Americans. As I mentioned earlier, "karoshi", a new phenomena, is occurring in Japanese culture. The man, generally, working every possible minute, going without sleep or any sort of home life, comes home late one night and drops over dead. He has in essence worked himself to death. We must begin to look at the roll of stress and sleep in our lives and our society, so that we can avoid karoshi here in this country.

When I was writing my book on PMS, I encountered a woman who blamed her symptoms on nuclear fallout. Although we may all laugh and feel she was exaggerating, on some levels she may in fact be right. There are numerous forms of environmental stress over which we have little control. Or at least, up until recently, we all believed were either irrelevant or unworthy of our attention. For instance, few of us realize that such things as poor air quality or acid rain are actually forms of toxic stress, as well as, possible forms of toxic poisoning. In other words, before toxic waste dumps and nuclear fallout kills us, it will definitely make us very nervous.

We must also look at other factors that control our environment, such as, smoke emanating from factories, industrial fumes, our own automobiles stuck in traffic for hours at a time, not to mention the exhalation of a chain smoker you happen to be trapped in the same room with or, for that matter, on the same planet with.

Then there is our food supply. Much of our food is contaminated in one way or another. Now some of you will argue with me and think I'm overreacting, but I'm not. We need to take a good, hard look at the kind of environmental stress that we have created in just the last 100 years. We now inject our animals with everything from steroids to antibiotics. We spray our food with chemicals that we not only injest, but seep down into the water table. Not to mention, that we consume foods and beverages ladened with artificial sweeteners and preservatives. In addition, we live with electromagnetic fields, and we are constantly bombarded with their effects by such things as electric blankets, televisions, microwave ovens and, of course, overhead power sources. Now, perhaps, any single item mentioned is not a threat by itself, but when you begin to add the cumulative effects of each of these facts to our body's ability to handle environmental stress, you can see the potential for disaster. In my opinion, our bodies have not been able to "catch up" environmentally with our ability to produce technology and new science. While it is all well and good to have ample sources of food available to people, and we all want the lights to go on when we flip the switch, we need to understand the long-term impact of these stresses on our sleep cycles and our mental well-being. All of the stresses that we have been talking about deplete the body of valuable supplies of the critical brain chemical, serotonin, without which we can not hope to sleep well and feel well.

There are differences in the way men and women experience stress. Women, in the past, were perceived as being the weaker sex. In other words, males have long seen women as being more vulnerable and easily stressed. Of course, we know this isn't true. Part of the reason women were viewed in this manner has to do with their brain chemistry and their menstrual cycle. Because the menstrual cycle uses up necessary brain serotonin during the luteal phase (second half), women are more prone to sleep deprivation than their male counterparts. Add to this, the fact that women require at least one hour more sleep than men, and you can see that means many women are experiencing severe symptoms associated with sleep deprivation. This sleep deprivation causes stress, and stress causes sleep deprivation, and on and on. Another interesting difference between men and women is that women have higher levels of toxic brain chemicals than do men. New research into the chemical make-up of tears indicates that tears, which are a result of sadness (versus tears that are a result of say cutting onions), differ in chemical make-up. It is believed by researchers that tears are the body's way of eliminating toxic brain chemicals. Thus, women cry more frequently than do men.

There are certainly differences in the way men and women communicate, and this difference is obvious to anyone who has ever felt frustration with communicating with members of the opposite sex. Women speak an average of 7000 words per day, while men only average 2000. These differences in communication styles can also add stress both in the working world and on the home front. Men tend to communicate in a more direct manner, whereas women tend to communicate in ways that are broader and envelope emotion.

New research indicates that women tend to actually have better "hard-wiring" between the right and left hemispheres of their brains. This may account for why many women have been labeled emotional or intuitive. Women tend to better at the "big picture", while men tend to be very focused. Perhaps, because initially women were gatherers and men were hunters. Of course, these are generalizations, and no one is exactly alike. As new research develops on brain function and communication techniques, we will hopefully be able to end the so called "war of the sexes". In addition to these problems, women have also had to contend with PMS, trying to be superwomen and balancing motherhood with the fast track.

The flip side of the coin is, of course, that things have not been that stress free for men either. Men, by nature, have testosterone levels that tend to make them more aggressive and competitive. In modern times, it isn't really necessary to hunt down our dinner and bring it home like the heroes of yesterday. So modern man has had to take his aggressions out at work, at the gym or on the golf course. Thus, the higher incidence of violence, frustration, stress-related disease and even criminal behavior. Even if a man is able to control these feelings, the stresses that are placed on him each day do nothing, but help put him in an early grave.

There are many things that we need to do to begin to live the kind of life that diminishes bad stress and enables us to utilize good stress. If I wanted to brain wash someone, I would first deprive them of normal sleep, and then I would instill some negative message, such as, you are worthless, you don't deserve to be successful, you always make mistakes, I can't count on you. When a person is experiencing stress and accompanying sleep deprivation, they will often have a negative attitude. From this negativity comes what I call, "down talk". In other words, the individual begins to self-program a negative self-image.

So how do we begin to overcome "down talk" and begin to program in "up talk"? The first step in any stress management program must include a complete sleep evaluation, diet and exercise. (More on this in later chapters.) The next step is what I call "priority planning", taking stock of what you can live with and what you can live without. I feel that in today's fast paced society, many of us have lost the ability to obtain quality life. So "quality control" must become part of

your stress reduction program. In addition to pri-
oritizing and looking at the quality of life, it is
also imperative to have the right attitude. The
right attitude can make the difference between
seeing your life as abundant and full versus
empty or meaningless. You can't have the right
attitude unless you sleep correctly and instill
positive messages to your subconscious. Some
of these attitude adjusters include affirmations.
An affirmation can include anything that you
would like. Some examples are "I am smart", "I
make good decisions", "people like me", etc. By
saying these things over and over in your mind,
as well as by writing them down, your unconscious brain begins to believe them causing them
to become true. Place some adhesive colored
dots on places that you see every day, such as
your review mirror, the mirror in the bathroom,
or the refrigerator, and each time you look at
them, think "relax", then notice if your body
feels tense. If you do feel tense, take a deep
breath, the kind that makes your abdomen move
outward, and think of your positive affirmations.
You can also program your mind in other positive ways. This is why hypnosis, meditation or
stress management tapes are so effective. If you
are in a semi-sleep state, such as hypnosis or
meditation, and you instill positive messages,

the unconscious side of your brain reacts as though these statements were, in fact, true. In other words, you become a "good decision maker", thought of by others and yourself as "smart", the kind of person "people like and respect". Hypnosis or meditation can be an invaluable tool in your fight for stress reduction.

It's often difficult to react in a positive way to negative situations encountered on a daily basis. For instance, I once had a superior whose management style was to get angry and make everyone as miserable as possible. Needless to say, she needed an attitude adjustment. However, my research has clearly shown that staying positive is often the best way to diffuse a negative situation. In other words, by taking responsibility for your own stress level, by sleeping, eating, exercising and reducing stress, you can become the kind of person who is positive and influences others to feel good about themselves. Often, in the beginning of a program such as this, it can be helpful to try to surround yourself with positive people. Have you ever noticed that those people who really are happy with themselves and have a great attitude are often like magnets drawing others to them? Eventually, even the negative individuals you encounter can be turned around.

The key is taking responsibility for yourself. Can you imagine a world where each person took responsibility for themselves and their well-being, rather than worrying about what someone else was doing? This reminds me of a sign I recently saw in a business establishment which read, "We are not responsible for our own errors". Although it was a joke, it often seems as though this has become a national slogan.

There have been plenty of studies which indicate that a positive attitude can impact your health and well-being on many levels. The effects have even been demonstrated on those who have been diagnosed as having a terminal illness. It is also becoming increasingly clear that increased sleep quality and quantity impacts the immune system in a positive way.

Find some stress reduction techniques that make you happy, and enjoy doing them. Perhaps, hypnosis (one of my personal favorites), guided visualization through stress reduction tapes, yoga, thai chi or other forms of exercise (I continue to love training with free weights, skiing is my new passion, and I've just started using a stairmaster). This year I am starting Yoga or Tai Chi. As of the writing of this book, I am 46 years old, and it's fun to find out that you're not too old to learn something new. My husband, Michael, and I learned to ski only four years ago, and it helped to save my sanity when I was going through the stresses of the last few years.

Plan time out for fun, either weekends away or at home, whatever you like. Whatever happened to having good, old-fashion fun. Invite friends over, and make it stress free - pot luck! Live as though it were the last day of your life, not the first. None of us know how much time we have, make the most of it TODAY. As my wise husband always says, "What difference is any of this going to make in a hundred years, anyway?"

And for heaven's sake, let's drop this he-man/ superwoman syndrome. After all, none of us are perfect, and we certainly have to stop and smell the roses sometime. Hopefully, we'll stop before our funeral! Too many men and women are living their lives as though it were a monopoly game. Let's see how much money and how many toys we can collect. Or let's try to be perfect, meet everyone's needs, but our own. After all, we're young or we were young, and we can have fun later, perhaps, when we retire. I'm not suggesting that you live unresponsibly, but that you decide what's important and what is not. I can tell you from personal experience that sleep

is one of the most important aspects of my life.
With quality sleep, I experience a life full of joy.
Without it, the same life appears dull and meaningless. So wake up, and make sleep the fuel to
improve your life—sleep matters!

STRESS TIPS

- Do some form of regular stress reduction daily—increase this during periods of stress.

- Experiment with different forms of stress reduction to find what is right for you.

- Regular body checks can be helpful in assessing your stress level.

- Place adhesive dots around your house to remind you to do these body checks.

- Try diaphramatic deep breathing—deep breaths that actually make your abdomen expand.

- Write or think positive affirmations daily.

- Never take on more stress than you can handle, say no when you mean no.

- Take ownership of your own wellness and attitude—you have the power and the tools to feel good every day.

- Remember sleep is the most important factor in eliminating stress.

- Learn, laugh and play daily—try new things, develop enthusiasm for life.

- Share your experiences with others.

- Plan ahead—this helps decrease stress.

- Prioritize—do the things that are the most important, eliminate those that are not.
- Never try to be all things to all people—do what is best for you.
- Avoid over-extending in all aspects of your life.
- Remember that in order to keep stress at a minimum—sleep matters!

8 Food For Thought

Learn to Sharpen Your Mind

Z Z Z Z Z Z Z Z Z Z Z Z Z Z Z Z Z Z Z Z Z Z Z Z Z Z

If you've read this far, you know that a good night's sleep is something you just can't take for granted. You know you need your sleep, you know you probably don't always get it, and you know that getting it isn't always that easy.

We've already looked at how little quality sleep most people get, and what actually constitutes quality sleep. What we haven't talked about is how you can get the kind of sleep you need. I cannot emphasize strongly enough my belief that the secret of getting a good night's sleep lies in what you eat. And I'm not talking about that piece of pizza you had before you went to bed that's keeping you awake, either. What I am talking about is a program of good nutrition coupled with a program of exercise, a program that is consistent and a program that allows for fun, as well as, relaxation.

During the past decade and a half, there has been so much talk about the serious shortage of oil, gasoline and other power sources, we've found it all too easy to avoid the inner energy crisis we have created within our own bodies.

By continuing to consume far more calories than we burn, we are conserving too much food energy as fat. While it's true that food is our greatest source of energy, food, in itself, can do nothing for us unless we actually put it to use and utilize it as energy.

In the beginning, of course, it was Mother Nature's way to hoard a little extra cache of goodies from the times of plenty, so we'd have something to fall back on during the hard times ahead. The trouble is, in today's society, few of us ever get to the kind of hard times that beleaguered our own rugged ancestors. Indeed, we're eating a lot more than the pioneers did and doing a lot less to work it off. As a result, many of us carry a residual load of unused fat with us wherever we go.

The latest surveys tell us that there are now more than 75 million overweight Americans. This is due not only to lack of physical exercise, but also to increased fat consumption in our diets.

Sugar consumption is another serious threat. If you don't believe that, here are some alarming statistics to change your mind. The average American consumes 125 pounds of sugar every year. That's about six ounces or close to 700 calories a day. Sadly, the answer, though, is not artificial sweeteners. As I mentioned in earlier chapters, many artificial sweeteners which contain phenylalinine also can cause serious problems with our blood brain barrier and our ability to convert the all-important amino acid, L-tryptophan, into serotonin, thus interfering with a good night's sleep. (See Appendix C.)

Too much salt in our diet is another growing problem. Oddly enough, salt was once so rare, it was used to pay off the military. Hence, the word salary. But, now it's so cheap and available, it is sprinkled on streets to melt the ice and snow. As a nearly universal presence in our processed food supply, salt is now one of our dietary villains.

Saturated fats, particularly the kind found in that big, fat, juicy steak, also increase the risk of degenerative diseases, notably heart disease. And high fat content has also been implicated in such diseases as colon cancer and breast cancer. The fat content in the average American diet now amounts to a whopping 40 percent of the calories consumed. That's not surprising when you remember that the fat in prime red meat can account for 50 to 70 percent of its calories. Many ranchers have started breeding leaner beef which is certainly a move in the right direction. However, when we really look at the kind of food shortages that exist in the world today, it seems ludicrous to continue to eat so much meat. When we consider that large amounts of meat are not only detrimental to our health, but also require so much more energy to produce.

I recently read that if our meat consumption was decreased by as little as 10 percent, there would be enough food in the world to feed every hungry person. I find this to be a staggering statistic, and one which I hope everyone will take seriously when they make their own food choices.

Another unfortunate food trend, fiber consumption has been cut in half since 1900. Its decline is accompanied by rising profits for the laxative industry. What happens when fiber is removed from foods and replaced by sugar and fat? The answer is alarming. For now, there are more calories per bite. Add to that, the growing concern of lower fiber diets and their implication in such diseases as colon cancer, and one can begin to appreciate the importance of a high fiber diet.

When we view the relationship between our food habits and our health status, then compare it to the more traditional patterns around the world, we come up with some surprising answers. For example, there are 20 population groups throughout the world where blood pressures don't rise with age, and hypertension simply doesn't exist. In each of these countries, the diets followed have not been significantly altered by Western standards. For the most part, the natives consume diets that are low in fat and sodium. But as soon as these people start adopting American food habits, their blood pressures go on the rise. Clearly, there is a lot at stake here.

But what we eat isn't necessarily the only critical factor in the way that our body metabolizes foods. It appears, after studying the French diet which is very high in animal fat, that perhaps the way we eat our food is also a critical factor. Too many Americans consume food on the run. In our harried pace to work 60 to 80 hours a week, we often don't stop and truly enjoy our food. We need to take time for conversation, relaxation and a few minutes to really allow our digestive system to work fully.

Health care costs have risen a staggering 1,000 percent plus over the last decade. And certainly, there is no way to measure the cost of this in human terms. The irony here is that never before has the relationship between nutrition and health been made so clear to the public. It appears that everyone is on some sort of food or diet regimen these days. But most people are having trouble sticking with it on any kind of a permanent basis.

Miraculously enough, we all inhabit bodies awesomely designed to offer us the best chance for survival with a scarce food supply. That's the good news. The bad news is that technology has given us more than we can eat. It's even more interesting to note that the human body has not changed appreciably since the days of Cro-Magnon man 35,000 years ago.

Then, as now, the body must have certain fuels in order to function well. These would include such things as adequate calories, protein (proteins are made of essential amino acids), fat, carbohydrates, vitamins, minerals and, of course, water. These needs have not changed. On the other hand, the food supply of Western man has changed more during the past 50 to 100 years than in all the tens of thousands of preceding years. In other words, our body's needs haven't changed, but the way we have chosen to fulfill these needs during the past half century or so, has changed dramatically. Add to this the kinds of changes that have been made in our water supply because of chemical contamination, our food supply which is constantly being sprayed with pesticides, our animal protein which is injected with everything from steroids to antibiotics, and you begin to see the kind of cumulative environmental impact that these substances are having on our nutritional status.

So the problem really becomes two-fold. First, there is the increase in fats and refined sugars which essentially act as empty calories. And second, we have chemical additives such as artificial sweeteners and the above mentioned pesticides, steroids, antibiotics, etc., which lower our body's nutritional status and wreak havoc on our sleep cycle. Our food supply is simply changing too rapidly for our body to adapt. The cumulative effect of all these changes can impact our mental, as well as, our physical health.

Urged on by such instinctive signals from the body, and supported by the enticements of our advertising and marketing culture, the affluent *everyman* makes food choices that are no longer his healthiest. The push and pull of thousands of attractively dramatized food messages urging us to eat as much gaily-packaged, junk food as we can has resulted in the kind of compulsive buying pressure that goes beyond our body's internal logic.

The fact that we have had a dramatic change in our eating habits relatively recently may also have had an influence on the sleep changes we are experiencing as a culture. As recently as 10,000 years ago, man was a hunter who ate game, fish, fowl and just about anything else he could catch. But he also ate roots, wild grains, fruits, fungus and berries. The first major change in his food supply came about 10,000 B.C. with the development of agriculture. It was then that the domestication of plants and animals enabled man to settle down. While this brought on some wonderful cultural advances, it really didn't alter his diet very dramatically, except to make it more secure.

From generation to generation, the human body has proven itself to be remarkably flexible and adaptable, always managing to make the best of whatever food supply happens to be available. But as I mentioned earlier, the body is best at conserving and meeting the challenges of a shortfall, since an extraordinary amount of any nutrients seems to lead to trouble.

It has also been observed that many standard, traditional foods are by no means harmless when taken in excess. For instance, there's a substance in potatoes called solanine which would reach toxic levels if 10 times the usual amount were eaten at one sitting. An unlikely situation to be sure, but one that could keep potatoes off the FDA's safe additives list. Other foods that are clearly nutritious, such as spinach and oatmeal, contain substances which interfere with the body's ability to make full use of some nutrients.

A lack of nutrients can also spell disaster. In some undeveloped countries, even today, there is a disease called "pellagra" which is usually brought on by a special kind of malnutrition. For one thing, in many of these poorer countries, the diets are based mainly on cornmeal which does not contain niacin or the all-important essential amino acid, L-tryptophan. It was when the natives of these countries were denied these essential amino acids that they began to develop this disease.

Among the symptoms are general nervousness, confusion, depression, apathy, delirium and severe sleep deprivation. Pellagra also affects women more than men, particularly those between the ages of 20 and 45. I found this to be particularly interesting because it appears that women in our own culture between these ages seem to be somewhat more susceptible to dietary and sleep changes than do others. This is probably due to the fact that menstruation actually uses up the brain chemical serotonin, so these women on a monthly basis are experiencing the kinds of brain chemical changes that make it more likely that they will experience changes in sleep patterns. When the pellagra patients were treated with L-tryptophan and vitamins all emotional symptoms, including sleep deprivation completely disappeared in a very short time.

It has always been clear that our diets and food habits are strongly linked to whatever emotional crisis we may be facing at any given time. We've all known of people who have overeaten because they are tired and want to increase their energy.

This can also be a similar excuse that's given for people who are drinking or are using recreational drugs. They may say they are using drugs or alcohol because they feel stressed, fatigued or depressed. However, these are not solutions to the problem at hand and, in fact, often intensify these symptoms.

One of the best preparations to meet our energy needs is a well-conditioned body. Conditioning can be achieved by keeping your weight down, indulging in a sensible amount of exercise and by modifying your intake of any of the dietary traps such as salt, sugar, artificial sweeteners, alcohol, drugs and tobacco.

I suppose I would summarize with a simple admonition to practice moderation when it involves any sort of dietary intake. Even more important, we should resist the temptation to think of food as being a form of recreation, or worse, as a method to reduce stress. Admittedly, when we consider the advertising input we receive daily, that kind of resistance grows more difficult every year.

The food marketing system is the largest user of national media advertising among all American industries. And more than three-quarters of their yearly budget is spent on pushing fun foods, or those of little or no nutritional value. The message the media gives us here is a kind of cultural reinforcement that matches the body's internal signals to eat sweets and fats.

So what kinds of food choices should we be making to ensure the best quality sleep possible? The importance of moderation in our dietary planning is critical. Learning to combine good nutrition, moderation and satisfying foods can offer a challenge. But the rewards of learning new ways to eat will benefit everyone. A sound program of good nutrition should include complex carbohydrates. (For a list of complex carbohydrates, please see the accompanying chart.) Somewhere between 60 to 70 percent of our daily calories should come from this source. Unfortunately, the American diet appears to be sorely lacking in complex carbohydrates, and it's too high in simple carbohydrates which are present in many refined foods. Complex carbohydrates are plentiful in all vegetables, fruits and whole grains such as rolled oats, brown rice, wheat and unsweetened cereals. They are also found in legumes, seeds, and nuts, as well as potatoes, breads and pasta. I highly recommend these foods be increased to a minimum of 60 percent and higher levels would be preferable. Protein should make up approximately 15 to 20 percent of the total caloric content of the food budget. The essential amino acids are found in complete proteins such as beef, fish, poultry, eggs, milk, yogurt and cheese. The body actually requires approximately 35 to 55 grams of protein per day or between 1 and 2 ounces. By increasing complex carbohydrates and decreasing protein, we can facilitate an increase in brain serotonin and improve the quality of our sleep (see diagrams 1, 2 & 3 on the following pages.) As I mentioned earlier, a 10% reduction in meat consumption could help to feed the entire world. I would like to suggest one meat-free day per week. This will help not only your health, but the rest of the planet as well.

It is also critical to reduce the amount of fat consumed. Calories derived from fat are, not only detrimental to health, but also rob the body of needed nutrients. Animal fat should be avoided whenever possible because it significantly raises cholesterol levels. Whenever possible, fat in the diet should be unsaturated, which means it does not contain cholesterol. The total percentage of fat in the diet should not be higher than 25 percent and lower if possible.

Diagram 3

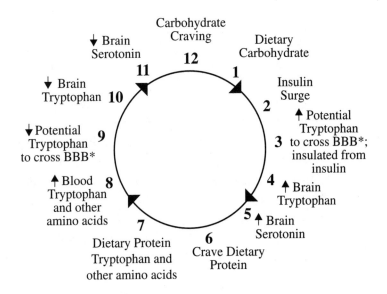

"Dietary Patterns"

1. Carbohydrate consumed.

2. Insulin surge secondary to carbohydrate consumption.

3. Tryptophan attaches itself to a protein molecule which insulates it from insulin. Other amino acids are unable to cross the blood-brain barrier in the presence of insulin. The competition for slots to cross the blood-brain barrier is decreased and more tryptophan crosses.

4. Increased levels of brain tryptophan occur.

5. Increased tryptophan allows increase in the brain serotonin.

6. Increased levels of brain serotonin cause cravings for dietary protein.

7. Dietary protein is consumed.

8. There is an increase in blood tryptophan and other amino acids.

9. Increased competition with other amino acids makes it more difficult for tryptophan to cross the blood-brain barrier.

10. Decreased brain tryptophan.

11. Decreased brain serotonin.

12. Carbohydrate craving, then consumption of dietary carbohydrate.

Diagram 4

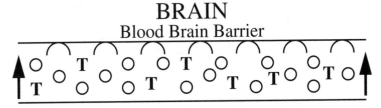

BRAIN
Blood Brain Barrier

○ = other amino acids trying to compete to cross the blood brain barrier and enter the brain

T = Tryptophan also trying to compete to enter the brain through the blood brain barrier

Diagram 5

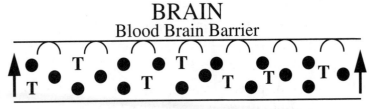

BRAIN
Blood Brain Barrier

● = other amino acids which have now become paralyzed in the presence of insulin and unable to compete to cross into the brain

T = Tryptophan; although there is no more tryptophan in the blood, because there is less competition, tryptophan can now cross easily. This will in turn make more tryptophan available and will increase brain serotonin.

Since it is often difficult to begin to make dietary changes, it is best to start gradually. Begin by adding additional, complex carbohydrates to your diet and reducing protein and fat slightly. Look at the positive effects these changes can make in your life and well-being and that of your family. Change takes time and patience. Try new foods whenever possible. Experiment a little, and try new taste sensations. Eat a wide variety of foods at each meal. Enjoy your food, eat more slowly and relax. View dinner with friends or family as a positive, enjoyable time. This will actually help enhance your body's ability to sleep better and stay healthy. Try to eat protein earlier in the day and complex carbohydrates later in the day. In other words, protein for breakfast and lunch, which makes you feel alert and energetic, and complex carbohydrates for dinner, which makes you feel calm, relaxed and helps you to sleep better. Avoid things like artificial sweeteners, caffeine, alcohol, preservatives, fat and salt in the diet.

Instead of viewing these dietary changes as a burden, look on them as a lifelong commitment to better health and better sleep. Remember—sleep matters!

Good Nutrition is essential for good health and enhancing sleep. Here are some helpful nutritional tips to help improve your sleep.

NUTRITIONAL TIPS

- Eat regular meals, chew your food well, and eat slowly.

- Relax and enjoy meal time.

- Plan regular meals and snacks.

- Take small portions, and eat only until you are comfortable.

- Increase whole grains, pasta, potatoes, brown rice and bread in your diet.

- Eat at least five servings of fruits and vegetables each day.

- Minimize animal protein and chose lean meats, poultry and fish.

- Avoid fat whenever possible, especially unsaturated fats.

- Avoid salt, learn to flavor your food with herbs and spices.

- Use less prepared and packaged foods.

- Read labels for fat content and additives, be aware of sodium, monosodium glutamate (MSG) and artificial sweetners and flavorings.

- Limit your sugar intake, but don't substitute with artificial sweetners.

- Try new foods, and eat a wide variety of foods.

- Whenever possible, eat with friends or family.

- Enjoy your food, and concentrate on what you are eating.

- Eat foods that you enjoy, providing they are nutritious.

- Use moderation in your consumption of alcohol and caffeine.

- Include vegetable sources of protein, such as dried peas, beans, nuts, seeds and tofu.

- Limit your use of eggs, organ meats, luncheon meats, sausage and bacon.

- Cook with less fat - bake, broil, roast, stew, barbecue or boil.

- Trim visible fat from meats.

- Avoid fad diets, instead exercise good nutritional judgment.

- Don't use food as a source of comfort.

- Never overeat.

- Expect that dietary changes take time; give yourself a break.

- Think of food as the fuel for your sleep cycle, your physical and mental health—sleep matters!

Diagram 5

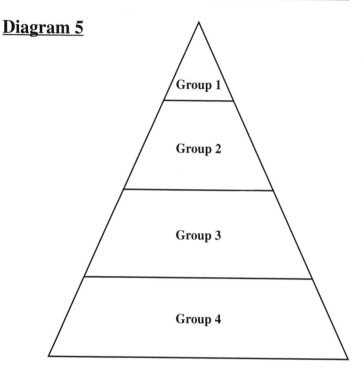

Group 1 - Foods to be eaten in very small amounts.

Group 2 - Foods to be eaten in very moderate amounts.

Group 3 - Foods to be eaten in moderation.

Group 4 - Foods to be eaten liberally - these should be the main stay of your diet.

GROUP 1

- Sweets
- Fats/oils
- Alcohol
- Preservatives
- Artificial Sweeteners

GROUP 2

- Whole Milk
- High fat cheeses
- Seeds/Nuts
- High fat meats
- Processed meats
- Charcoal broiled meats

GROUP 3

- Lowfat milk
- Yogurt
- Cheese
- Eggs
- Lean Meats
- Fish
- Poultry

GROUP 4

- Dark green and yellow fruits and vegetables
- Vitamin C-rich fruits and vegetables
- All other fruits and vegetables
- Legumes (dried beans and peas)
- Whole grains, breads, cereals, rice, pasta
- All forms of potatoes

9   *EZZZ - Living*

Get the Best Rest of Your Life

Z Z Z Z Z Z Z Z Z Z Z Z Z Z Z Z Z Z Z Z Z Z Z Z Z Z

Now that you know about the importance of good eating habits for sleep, let's take a look at other factors in your lifestyle and your immediate surroundings that may work for or against getting a good night's rest.

With that in mind, I've developed a sleep hygiene program which I believe is a sure-fire recipe for healthful sleep. It's based, not only on my own personal experience, but on the experience of my clients and findings by prominent sleep researchers, as well. These sleep strategies, many of them devised specifically for people with serious sleep disorders, should be useful for anyone who is having difficulty getting their sleep.

Many features of my program might seem pretty obvious at first glance, but just because they make sense doesn't mean you are necessarily following them. Your participation should begin many hours before it's time for you to retire.

Make sleep your first priority. Think of sleep as the greatest gift you can receive. And remember, no matter how convinced you may be that sleep is important, there are always plenty of distractions to get in the way of sleep. Unless it's an emergency, don't let anything interfere with following this program until you've tried it.

Talk about your sleep needs. Take the time to discuss what works for you with your immediate family, and ask them to let you know what works for them. Learn to respect their own sleep needs, as well. Friends and fellow workers can also provide you with valuable insights. You'll be surprised how many people are eager to talk about their sleep experiences. Only, they don't often get the chance because sleep isn't normally considered to be a suitable subject of conversation.

Control your intake. I've said it before, and I'll say it again. Avoid large amounts of coffee, tea or soft drinks that contain caffeine, especially late in the day. Even decaffeinated coffee can act as a stimulant for some sensitive people. Nicotine is another stimulant to be avoided.

Artificial sweeteners in "diet" products may affect your sleep, as well. Studies show that sugar substitutes such as aspartame, the "miracle" sweetener that's replaced sugar in so many food products, actually blocks the body's production of serotonin which, as I showed earlier, is a necessary precursor in the body's progression to sleep.

Eating a heavy meal in the evening or taking too much liquid in the late afternoon can agitate your digestive action and cause bladder discomfort. Instead, eat a light, protein-rich breakfast and lunch to encourage daytime alertness, and schedule dinner four to five hours before bedtime. And make it high in complex carbohydrates.

Get your exercise. Try to engage in some form of physical activity every day. Walking, for example, has been shown to be a remarkably effectively stimulus to successful sleep, and swimming is an excellent muscle relaxant. Aerobic exercise and weight training are also important for overall fitness. If you're a real fitness enthusiast whose regimen includes a strenuous workout, start by incorporating it into your late afternoon schedule. While this may clearly be impossible for most people, it's well worth considering as a way of relieving pent-up nervous energy brought on by the stresses of the day.

Remember that intensive physical exercise, and resulting muscle fatigue, don't necessarily equate with making it easier to fall asleep and stay asleep. If you engage in strenuous exercise (which has been proven to have negative effects on your metabolic equilibrium) too near the time you retire, you're risking being far too stressed and exhausted to insure adequate sleep.

Sometimes, a siesta is in order. Here, I'd like to take exception to the conventional wisdom concerning what I consider to be an indispensable component of any healthful sleep program, namely the much-maligned, afternoon nap. For some reason, probably having to do with our society's pervasive anti-sleep bias, some sleep experts have not recognized the value of naps. However, scientists who study biological clocks (they're known as chronobiologists) tell us that there's a natural urge to go to sleep late in the afternoon. So why not take advantage of it? Personally, I'm a strong believer in the institution,

and I've never known an afternoon nap to interfere with my ability to get a good night's sleep.

If you do take a nap, my advice is to go all out.
In other words, take off your clothes and get into
bed. In this respect, I have at least one historical
figure to back me up. When Winston Churchill,
whose legendary ability to cat-nap during the
Battle of Britain has been widely noted, was
asked for tips on napping, the famous British
statesman replied that he always tried to get out
of his clothes and get into bed when he took a
nap.

Keep in mind that naps can be of various kinds
and duration. While most of us can benefit physically from just a few minutes of rest, that
doesn't make lying down for a while any substitute for sleep. The body needs rest, but the brain
needs sleep. So the adage goes. And only when
your brain is rested, are you rested yourself.

Take time to unwind. Stretching exercises and
meditation techniques can help you get rid of the
tension that accumulates during the day. Earlier,
I discussed how proper sleep habits can enhance
the quality of your sex life, but the reverse is also
true. If healthy, safe sex is part of your life,
you'll sleep better for it.

Chill out. I'm a firm believer in hot baths, and not just because a soak in the tub is wonderfully relaxing. Studies show that one critical component of the sleep process is a drop in body temperature. That's exactly what happens after you bathe. This should be done at least one to two hours before retiring to allow the body time to cool down. By the same token, keep the bedroom cool, but not too cool. If room temperature is down around 50 degrees, you may tend to have disruptive dreams. Above 70 degrees, and there's a good chance you'll end up waking and thrashing around.

Make your wishes known. Write to your legislatures and the media, and let them know that you want the amino acid, L-tryptophan, returned to the market. Demand that the Food and Drug Administration regulate this amino acid in a way that will insure it's safety and the safety of other products on the market, so we will never have the kind of contamination that caused L-tryptophan to be removed from the market in the first place. (See Appendix B.)

Make your bed work for you. Whether you're taking a nap or going to sleep for the night, pay close attention to the specifics of your sleep environment. You'll never get a good night's rest if your bed isn't comfortable. The best mattress you can afford is probably one of the most important investments you'll ever make, especially when you take into account how much time you spend on it. Remember that even a good mattress has outlived its usefulness after ten years or so, and pillows should be replaced every few years.

As for bedding, I personally wouldn't be without my down comforter (down fill has beneficial electrostatic properties). And unless you sleep alone, you should have a king-size bed.

Pull the shades. A key factor in making your sleep metabolism work for you is darkness. As I discussed in an earlier chapter, our biological clock, the one that tells us when to go to sleep, takes its clues from the amount of light entering the optic nerve (that strategic portion of the brain which is responsible for producing the sleep-inducing chemical, melatonin—see Appendix C). This tiny area of the brain works in concert with the pineal gland to pour melatonin into the bloodstream, but bright light shuts off production of this key hormone.

For that reason alone, you need to insure that you're in the dark as much as possible when you go to sleep. It takes a sharp contrast in light and dark to trigger the conversion of serotonin to melatonin, which is the basic mechanism of sleep. We all require a vivid changeover from light to dark to get to sleep quickly and to insure the quality of sleep we need. Now check the blinds on your bedroom window. Do they block out street lights and the headlights of passing cars? And use a sleep mask if necessary. I do. (See order form in back of book.) Even the best blinds aren't designed to block out daytime light. So, if your schedule makes it imperative to sleep late, wear a sleep mask or have your bedroom fitted with blackout curtains. If you're disturbed by noises at night, try wearing ear plugs or purchasing a white noise device. Then, as soon as you're awake, draw the curtains and get plenty of sunlight or bright light.

On the other hand, you can put sleep metabolism to work for you by using sunlight to reset your body clock. Say you're not getting to sleep until 4 am, then sleeping in until noon. Get up an hour earlier than usual and sit outside. Natural light will cue your internal clock that the day is starting an hour earlier. After a few days of this, your body should adjust to the new time schedule.

Stick to your personal schedule. Don't let the time you go to sleep vary more than an hour earlier or two hours later than is comfortable for you. As I mentioned earlier, our body clock is set for 25 hours rather than 24 hours. Thus, we tend to want to go to bed later each night. If you want to take a nap before or after dinner, fine, but don't go to bed for the night too much before or after your regular sleep time. Go to bed at the same time each night and, even more important, try to get up at the same time each morning.

Cure bad sleep habits. Many people suffer from what experts call "conditioned insomnia". To put it bluntly, these people have acquired a lot of bad sleep habits. Look for danger signs in your sleep patterns. If you wake up within an hour or so of falling asleep, you may be too anxious or too overstimulated to go back to sleep immediately. If you still haven't fallen back to sleep after 20 or 30 minutes, get up, take a few minutes to attend to some unfinished chore, and, only then, go back to bed. If you still can't get to sleep, repeat the exercise until you finally do sleep. But still try to get up at the same time you've set yourself in the morning. Take a nap in the afternoon to help you catch up.

Get in the mood. Make your bedroom a haven from everyday worries and cares. Establish a sleep routine. If you eat a light snack at night, make sure it's a carbohydrate. And eat it at least two hours before retiring. Do not watch television in bed or try to do paperwork. If you're concerned about the following day's events, set aside some "worry time". Before you go to bed, make a chronological list of the next day's plans and projects on a fresh sheet of paper. Even if you keep a daily engagement calendar, your priorities can get jumbled. Put any relevant notes in order, and let your subconscious take over. Do the same things, in the same order before you go to bed. This will signal your subconscious that it's time to begin to fall asleep.

Don't toss and turn. One of the most effective ways of dealing with sleep loss may seem the most contradictory. "Sleep restriction" is the term used for reducing the ratio of hours you spend in bed to the hours you sleep on an average night. Simply stated, if you're having trouble falling asleep at night, stay up. The worst thing you can do is lie in bed trying to fall asleep. If you haven't fallen asleep within 20 or 30 minutes after going to bed, you should get up, go into another room and return only when you're tired enough to go to sleep. Try to finish a few tasks that keep you moderately active or alert.

Get enough sleep. One of the first steps in evaluating your need for sleep, not surprisingly, is to figure out how much sleep you actually get. A good night's rest and a little simple arithmetic will tell you how much sleep you need. Start by keeping track of what time you fell asleep and what time you wake up. If the amount of sleep you need is significantly more or less than eight and a half to ten hours, you're the exception.

If you need an alarm clock to wake you up, many experts suggest that you adjust your clock forward by 15 minutes a night until you find the amount of sleep that enables you to feel best throughout the day.

Whatever you do, don't short yourself on sleep. I believe people who have sufficient sleep are so much more effective at work. It's worth the extra time they spend sleeping.

Avoid sleep medication. When falling asleep becomes a preoccupation, many people resort to sedatives. Ironically, studies have shown that people who take sleeping pills after they can't sleep for a couple of hours, often fall asleep

instantly, well ahead of the time it takes a hyp-
notic drug to have any measurable physiological
effect. These people seem to find the mere act of
taking a pill so reassuring that the medication
could even be said to function, in effect, as a placebo. In other words, try to find other ways of
getting to sleep rather than relying on brand
name drugs with their accompanying risk of
unfortunate side effects. If you're already taking
some form of medication for sleep, talk with
your doctor about the possibility of tapering off
the medication slowly. DO NOT STOP ANY
MEDICATION ON YOUR OWN. CHECK
WITH YOUR DOCTOR AND BE SAFE.
Abrupt changes in your metabolism produced by
rapid withdrawal may make you feel an
increased urge to take the same medication.

Learn from *feng shui*. This venerable Chinese
discipline is dedicated to "the art of a harmoni-
ous environment". While some of the claims
made for *feng shui* may sound hard to believe,
there are many practical aspects of this ancient
tradition that make very good sense to me. For
example, *feng shui* masters believed you should
position your bed so you are facing the bedroom
doorway. It was thought that this arrangement
created an unconscious feeling of security. Also

eliminate any clutter from your bedroom. Stacks of magazines and newspapers, for example, are a subliminal source of distraction and uneasiness. If you wish to learn more, there are several popular books on the subject which will serve as an introduction.

Get professional help. If you think that sleep loss may be posing a serious threat to your emotional or physical well-being, you may want to seek out a therapist who can recommend specific cognitive techniques aimed at reducing your fears and insecurities. For example, some elderly people experience insomnia because they are secretly afraid of dying in their sleep. Less dramatic, but severely troublesome, are the many people suffering from insomnia who are caught in a vicious circle where they lie awake worrying about how their lack of sleep could affect their performance the following day. In addition, talk with your doctor or practitioner about your sleep problems. If he or she thinks it is necessary, ask for a referral to a sleep clinic in your area. They can evaluate your sleep complaints, and work with your doctor or practitioner to offer suggestions for your specific needs. (For a list, see Appendix A.)

Practice prudent avoidance. Finally, I should mention the presence of other even more subtle factors than those I've listed above which may also influence the quality of your sleep.

Take electromagnetic radiation, for example. Until recently, there has been limited public awareness of the potential health threats from electrical power supplies, but researchers are now increasingly concerned about the effects of the magnetic component of electrical power on human health. My advice would be to follow the suggestions of governmental studies which advocate "prudent avoidance" of exposure to electrical fields.

You can easily accomplish this by keeping a safe distance from electrical gadgets, such as the ever present alarm clock. And if you feel you have to use an electric blanket, try turning the thermostat on half an hour or so before you get into bed, then turn it off when you do retire.

So now you're sound asleep. What happens next? Earlier I talked about the nightly drama of sleep. What you do with that makes for a fascinating story, and the subject of the following chapter.

Sleep is the Key to eliminating emotional ups and downs. It's critical to your state of mind and your physical health that you develop good sleep habits—sleep matters!

EZZZ—LIVING TIPS

- If you're chronically tired, see your doctor to make sure you don't have a medical problem.

- Give yourself at least a day a week when you can get an extra hour or two of sleep.

- Keep track of your activities and see where you can increase your sleep time - perhaps you can turn off the TV an hour earlier.

- Develop regular sleep habits and stick to them.

- Sleep a minimum of eight hours per night, longer if you need it.

- Sleep in a dark, quiet and cool room.

- Invest in a comfortable, firm mattress.

- Make sleep time a high priority in your life.

- Discuss the importance of sleep with other family members.

- Minimize sleep interruptions.

- Take naps - 15 minutes to two hours can be refreshing

- Eat a well balanced diet.

- Exercise in the afternoon; whenever possible, avoid late night exercise.

- Develop a sleep routine before bedtime.
- Unwind prior to trying to fall asleep with an activity such as reading, TV or a hot bath—something you find relaxing.
- Practice some form of regular stress reduction.
- Awaken to bright lights by turning on lights and opening drapes in the morning.
- Wash your face or shower upon arising to help you wake up.
- Avoid altering your sleep schedule more than one hour early or two hours later than your usual bed time.
- Avoid sleep medications, tranquilizers or antihistamines to help you sleep - DO NOT STOP THESE MEDICINES IF YOU ARE CURRENTLY TAKING THEM WITHOUT YOUR DOCTORS PERMISSION AND SUPERVISION.
- Don't drink large amounts of alcohol; an occasional drink is OK (moderation is the key here).
- Moderation is also important in coffee and cola drinks prior to bed.
- Avoid nicotine - stop smoking.
- Do NOT use artificial sweeteners.

- Avoid long drives or dangerous chores when you are extremely sleep deprived.
- ABOVE ALL, HAVE A GOOD NIGHT'S SLEEP, YOU DESERVE IT!

10 *Night School*

Make Your Dreams Come True

Z Z Z Z Z Z Z Z Z Z Z Z Z Z Z Z Z Z Z Z Z

Now that I've demonstrated the importance of healthful sleep and showed you how to make sure you get it, this is a good time to talk about a creative approach to maximizing your sleep potential. In a previous chapter, we looked at the marvelously, intricate and subtle structure of sleep, as reflected in the continuous progression from deep sleep to dream state. But what actually happens during the time we spend dreaming?

Since the dawn of recorded history, dreams have been the subject of much awe and speculation. They've been regarded by poets and philosophers as valuable clues to the interpretation of present and future events. But in modern times, the signs and symbols of dreams were relegated to the realm of psychoanalysis. Dreams were seen as evidence of some underlying neurosis, a mind set that probably helped contribute to what I see as a popular denial of the validity of dreams. Contributing to this perception, the dreams most people seem to remember, if they remember them at all, are usually "bad" ones. It's a small wonder that many of us operate in a form of dream denial, and as a result, are often nervous and evasive about their dreams. "I had the craziest dream last night," someone will say, as if dream content is only a matter of amusement. Dreams are similarly linked, in the popular imagination, to horror movies on late-night television or blamed on indigestion.

It may surprise you to learn that this dismissive view of dreams is no longer considered to be especially scientific. In recent years, sleep researchers who look carefully at the dream process have come to some startling conclusions about the role of dreams in our daily lives. And while much of this information comes from scientific studies, some of the most profound discoveries about dream function originate in the investigations of anthropologists who have examined the dream life of one of the world's most primitive tribes.

One day while I was beginning work on this book, a colleague of mine who knew I was interested in dream theory asked me if I'd ever heard of an obscure, Malaysian hill tribe known as the Senoi. According to my friend, the Senoi are a primitive people who had only recently been studied in any depth by anthropologists. What the scientists who visited with the Senoi had discovered sounded truly remarkable.

"The Senoi were different from surrounding tribes," my friend told me. They lived at peace with themselves and with their neighbors who, in turn, expended much time and energy waging war against each other. An exceptionally creative people, the Senoi spent much of their time engaged in artistic pursuits. The Senoi were remarkable in other respects. Individually, they appeared to possess a level of psychological maturity unlike anything previously observed in other primitive or modern societies. "Compared to the Senoi," my friend told me, "most Westerners are stuck in a preadolescent stage of psychological development."

The Senoi, it turned out, placed enormous significance on their dream life. Every morning, over the first meal of the day, family members compared dreams they remembered from the night before. Children were encouraged to describe their dreams in detail, and their elders took turns explaining what they meant. Afterwards, the adults left their dwellings for a village meeting where, once again, their dreams of the previous night were also discussed. It was on the basis of these dreams that plans for important village matters were decided.

I found my friend's account very interesting, of course. After all, sleep and dreams were a major concern in my work. But what did the superstitions of a primitive Malaysian hill tribe have to do with me? "The Senoi also have a basic script they are encouraged to follow in their dreams," my friend continued. "In this scenario, there are three main dramatic actions."

"During sleep, you first confront one or more dream figures who represent some kind of physical threat or danger. Second, you fight them off. Third, after you have confronted them, you subdue them and force them to give you a gift. The final resolution comes after you wake, when you ask for and receive recognition from your family and peers that the gift you obtained was valuable."

All well and good, I thought, but I couldn't help wondering what the "scenario" my friend described had to do with me. As I've mentioned, I knew my dream experiences had some major implications for me personally. My "baby dream" was proof enough of that (more on this later). But, the Senoi scenario seemed completely foreign to my own dream patterns.

However, that same night I had exactly the dream my friend described. I was confronted with a threatening dream figure, I fought him off, I demanded a gift, I was given it. Now, I'm well aware that I am probably fairly suggestible where sleep and dreams are concerned. After all, sleep and dreams are part of my job. But, the Senoi dream pattern has continued to repeat itself, even on occasions when I've taken a long nap.

What's doubly interesting to me about my initiation into these so-called "primitive" dream patterns is the effect that Senoi dreaming has had on my own life. At the time I first became acquainted with the way that the Senoi dream, I was facing enormous personal challenges in my career. As I mentioned earlier, I had written a book about the role of L-tryptophan in the treatment of premenstrual syndrome which I published myself and extensively promoted, only to be confronted with a disastrous turn of events that effectively stalled my prospects for success.

In the process, I'd been thwarted by my book distributor, I was involved in a traumatic legal altercation with an entrepreneur who was supposed to be paying me to market a line of formulations for PMS but who had embroiled me in costly litigation over the profits, and I had quit my job as a physician's assistant. Luckily, my personal life was back on track. Thanks to the control I'd won over PMS, I had my family back, and I now had the loving support of my husband and daughter. Professionally, however, my life was a mess.

For a long time, I felt out of control and unable to make a decision about my future. In a sense, I think I felt completely defeated, and my dream life reflected this sense of defeat. However, after I began to dream in the manner of the Senoi, I began to slowly regain my sense of self. The difference for me was that now, in my dreams at least, I was fighting back and being rewarded for it.

As it turns out, my experience with the Senoi way of dreaming was not all that different from the modern practice of lucid dreaming. It now appears that our dreams, or so many sleep experts are convinced, are instrumental in reinforcing a sense of self-esteem that appears to be essential to healthy psychological functioning. Furthermore, they tell us, we can actively participate in our dream life in a way that can have long lasting psychological advantages.

It seems to me that, while the current model of lucid dreaming is fine as far as it goes, the resolution that comes during lucid dreaming must occur in the final REM stage of sleep. Since we seldom have the opportunity to recall the contents of earlier dream stages during the night, I suspect that elements of conflict characterize these preparatory dream states.

It may even be true that, without an understanding of how and why we dream or how to go about determining the outcome of our dreams, we can never attain full psychological maturity. If that is indeed the case, then I don't think it's too farfetched to speculate that our limited awareness of the contribution that dreams offer could even explain much of what is wrong with contemporary society.

As it turns out, some sleep researchers have identified a previously unrecognized dynamic in the dream schedule, involving three to four distinct stages of decision-making and conflict resolution which manifest themselves as dream "scenarios". According to one leading proponent of lucid dreaming, these serial dreams help us to complete a kind of emotional "homework".

These dreams occur in stages which, to continue the learning metaphor, are referred to as "the three R's," with "a fourth R" that emerges when we are under unusual stress. According to this model, the first dream of the night constitutes a "review" of who we are (the first "R"), followed by a dream to "revise" our concept of self (the second "R"), then by a dream that allows us to "rehearse" our revised concept of self (the third "R") and help us prepare for where we are going. When we suffer from undue stress in our lives, the dream process intervenes with a mechanism for repair (the fourth "R"). Given the stressful nature of modern lives, I would expect that this fourth dream phase would occur fairly frequently during sleep. That is, if we allowed ourselves to sleep long enough to reap the benefits and repair our stresses.

As you can see, science has come a long way in recent years in so far as our appreciation of the importance of dreams is concerned. But I wonder if researchers aren't still missing another important clue to their function. I'm referring, again, to the metabolic pathways of sleep, particularly as they concern the conversion of tryptophan to serotonin and then to melatonin (see Appendix C). I don't think it's unreasonable to suggest that these fundamental biochemical processes are somehow reflected in the conflict and resolution scenarios that proponents of lucid dreaming describe.

At this writing, I don't know of any studies linking sleep metabolism to a satisfactory dream life, but the connection would seem to be a promising one for future dream research. Some experts on lucid dreaming are already saying that biochemical transformations during sleep are reflected in our dreams. And that our dreams may function as signposts in such basic physiological functions as the healing process, but so far the importance of the pathways to serotonin conversion apparently hasn't aroused much curiosity in the scientific community. Which brings me back to my 'baby dream'. I remember vividly the night I dreamt about a beautiful pink baby I was holding in my arms some 27 years ago. I knew in my heart, I had conceived. It was only a few weeks later, I found out that I was pregnant with my daughter, Jill. I have heard others tell of similar incidents. Our subconscious mind knows what is occurring in our body and can tell us of both impending danger and good fortune. The body's ability to signal warning signs of our risk of accidents, illness and other major life changes is well documented.

This lack of research is a glaring omission as far as I'm concerned. And while I'm confident that this will change as new scientific evidence comes to light, in the meantime, any argument for the contribution of serotonin and the amino acid L-tryptophan in lucid dreaming must be based on insight and intuition. My own experience and the experience of several thousand others who have taken this amino acid has clearly shown an increase in the awareness of dreams. When I first started taking this product, I began to dream vivid dreams, often in color with intricate plots. Initially, my dream life was so vivid that it was almost frightening. I have since learned that REM rebound is a common occurrence in those who have been chronically deprived of REM sleep. When the body is finally given the chemicals it needs to facilitate normal sleep, it must respond in this way. After the first week or two, my dream life, and that of my patients became much richer.

AGAIN, DO NOT TAKE L-TRYPTOPHAN UNTIL THE FDA RELEASES IT BACK ON THE MARKET. (For information on where to write see the address in the back of this book.)

While your metabolism is working to repair your dreams, you can also put your conscious awareness of what you dream to work for you. Of course, if you're like most people, you probably aren't used to remembering much of what you dream, but you can change that, too.

You can take the first step in remembering your dreams before you go to sleep. As simple as it may sound, you need to make a deliberate effort to tell yourself to remember at this time.

Everyone dreams, usually half a dozen times a night that is if you're getting an adequate amount of sleep time in. People who say they don't dream aren't lying, exactly, they just don't remember that they've dreamed. Their notion that they don't dream is merely an indication that they're not waking up at the appropriate stage of sleep.

The most important thing to know about remembering your dreams is that when you awaken naturally, meaning, when you are fully rested and ready to wake up, you will awaken immediately from a dream. As I mentioned in an earlier chapter, the "morning dream" is the longest dream, sometimes lasting a half to three quarters of an hour, during an uninterrupted night of sleep. Research has shown that natural sleepers wake up directly following this last REM stage of sleep.

Five minutes after REM stops, your dream recall is fragmentary at best; ten minutes after, recall is almost completely gone. So the first rule in remembering your dreams is: Don't use an alarm clock or any other artificial stimulus to make yourself wake up, or you may miss this crucial dream period.

Now that you've set the stage for total dream recall, keep the following strategies in mind (especially while you're drifting off to sleep).

As you wake up, keep your eyes closed, lie still, and let your thoughts drift. If you still can't recall your dream, try the same random thought strategy I suggested in my earlier chapter about getting to sleep.

Until now, you have remained lying still. When you've triggered your initial dream recall and feel satisfied, you can command further remembering by the simple strategy of shifting your position in bed. When you feel you've recalled all you can of your dream to this point, keeping your eyes closed, gradually shift to another position where you feel comfortable. Most likely this will be another position you maintained earlier while you dreamed. For reasons that are not clearly understood, repeating the same position will help trigger further recall of your dreams.

Once you've learned how to recall your dreams, you may be interested in recording them. Some authors have published detailed suggestions about how to do just this. But, for general purposes, I feel it is more important for you to wake with an awareness of your dreams, and to feel good about them. Just remember, anything you can bring with you from your dreams into your waking life is all to the good, especially if you can share your dreams with friends. Above all, keep in mind that the more significance you attach to your dreams, the easier you will find them to remember.

Enhancing your sleep and dreams can benefit you in more ways than you can imagine.

Improved mood, personal happiness and a positive mental outlook are only some of the rewards of a good night's sleep. Sweet dreams!

Appendix A

Listing of Sleep Clinics

Z Z Z Z Z Z Z Z Z Z Z Z Z Z Z Z Z Z Z Z Z Z Z

The following sleep disorders programs are accredited members of the American Sleep Disorders Association. You can obtain a current listing and additional information by writing, The National Sleep Foundation, 1367 Connecticut Avenue, NW, Suite 200, Washington, DC 20036.

*Accredited as Specialty Laboratory for Sleep Related Breathing Disorders. All other programs are accredited Full Service Sleep Disorders Centers.

Sleep Disorders Center
Providence Hospital
3200 Providence Drive
PO Box 196604
Anchorage, AK 99519-6604

Sleep Disorders Center of Alabama, Inc.
790 Montclair Road, Suite 200
Birmingham, AL 35213

Brookwood Sleep Disorders Center
Brookwood Medical Center
2010 Brookwood Medical Center Drive
Birmingham, AL 35209

Sleep-Wake Disorders Center
University of Alabama at Birmingham
1713 6th Avenue South
CPM Building, Room 270
Birmingham, AL 35233-0018

Sleep-Wake Disorders Center
Flowers Hospital
4370 West Main Street, PO Box 6907
Dothan, AL 36302

Hunstville Hospital Sleep Disorders Center
101 Sivley Road
Huntsville, AL 35801

Alabama North Regional Sleep Disorders Center
250 Chateau Drive, Suite 235
Huntsville, AL 35801

Southeast Regional Center for Sleep/Wake Disorders
Springhill Memorial Hospital
3719 Dauphin Street
Mobile, AL 36608

Sleep Disorders Center
Mobile Infirmary Medical Center
PO Box 2144
Mobile, AL 36652

USA Knollwood Sleep Disorders Center
University of South Alabama Knollwood Park Hospital
5600 Girby Road
Mobile, AL 36693-3398

Baptist Sleep Studies Laboratory*
Baptist Medical Center
2105 East South Boulevard
Montgomery, AL 36116-2498

Tuscaloosa Clinic Sleep Lab*
701 University Boulevard East
Tuscaloosa, AL 35401

Pediatric Sleep Disorders
Arkansas Children's Hospital
800 Marshall Street
Little Rock, AR 72202-3591

Sleep Disorders Center
Baptist Medical Center
9601 I-630, Exit 7
Little Rock, AR 72205-7299

Desert Samaritan Sleep Disorders Center
Desert Samaritan Medical Center
1400 South Dobson Road
Mesa, AZ 85202

Sleep Disorders Center
Good Samaritan Medical Center
1111 East McDowell Road
Phoenix, AZ 85006

Sleep Disorders Center at Scottsdale Memorial Hospital
Scottsdale Memorial Hospital-North
10450 North 92nd Street
Scottsdale, AZ 85261-9930

Appendix A

Sleep Disorders Center
University of Arizona
1501 North Campbell Avenue
Tucson, AZ 85724

WestMed Sleep Disorders Center
1101 South Anaheim Boulevard
Anaheim, CA 92805

Mercy Sleep Laboratory*
Mercy San Juan Hospital
6501 Coyle Avenue
Carmichael, CA 95608

Downey Community Hospital Sleep Disorders Center
Rio Hondo Foundation Hospital
8300 East Telegraph Road
Downey, CA 90240

Palomar Medical Center Sleep Disorders Lab*
Palomar Medical Center
555 East Valley Parkway
Escondido, CA 92025

Sleep Disorders Institute
St. Jude Medical Center
100 East Valencia Mesa Drive
Suite 308
Fullerton, CA 92635

Glendale Adventist Medical Center Sleep Disorders
Center
Glendale Adventist Medical Center
1509 Wilson Terrace
Glendale, CA 91206

Sleep Disorders Center
Scripps Clinic and Research Foundation
10666 North Torrey Pines Road
La Jolla, CA 92037

Sleep Disorders Center
Grossmont District Hospital
PO Box 158
La Mesa, CA 92044-0300

Respiratory Sleep Laboratory*
Antelope Valley Hospital Medical Center
1600 West Avenue J
Lancaster, CA 93534

Memorial Sleep Disorders Center
Long Beach Memorial Medical Center
2801 Atlantic Avenue
PO Box 1428
Long Beach, CA 90801-1428

Sleep Disorders Center
Cedars-Sinai Medical Center
8700 Beverly Boulevard
Los Angeles, CA 90048-1869

UCLA Sleep Disorders Center
Department of Neurology
710 Westwood Plaza
Los Angeles, CA 90024

North Valley Sleep Disorders Center
11550 Indian Hills Road
Suite 291
Mission Hills, CA 91345

Sleep Disorders Center
Hoag Memorial Hospital Presbyterian
301 Newport Boulevard
PO Box 6100
Newport Beach, CA 92658-6100

Sleep Evaluation Center
Northridge Hospital Medical Center
18300 Roscoe Boulevard
Northridge, CA 91328

California Center for Sleep Disorders
3012 Summit Street
5th Floor, South Building
Oakland, CA 94609

St. Joseph Hospital Sleep Disorders Center
1310 West Stewart Drive
Suite 403
Orange, CA 92668

Sleep Disorders Center
UC Irvine Medical Center
101 City Drive South
Orange, CA 92668

Sleep Disorders Center
Huntington Memorial Hospital
100 West California Boulevard
PO Box 7013
Pasadena, CA 91109-7013

Sleep Disorders Center
Doctors Hospital - Pinole
2151 Appian Way
Pinole, Ca 94564-2578

Pomona Valley Hospital Medical Center
Sleep Disorders Center
1798 North Garey Avenue
Pomona, CA 91767

Sleep Disorders Center
Sequoia Hospital
170 Alameda de las Pulgas
Redwood City, CA 94062-2799

Sleep Disorders Center at Riverside
Riverside Community Hospital
4445 Magnolia, E1
Riverside, CA 92501

Sutter Sleep Disorders Center
650 Howe Avenue
Suite 910
Sacramento, CA 95825

Mercy Sleep Disorders Center
Mercy Health Care San Diego
4077 Fifth Avenue
San Diego, CA 92103-2180

San Diego Sleep Disorders Center
1842 Third Avenue
San Diego, CA 92101

Sleep Disorders Center
California Pacific Medical Center
PO Box 7999
San Francisco, CA 94120-7999

Sleep Disorders Center
San Jose Medical Center
675 East Santa Clara Street
San Jose, CA 95112

Santa Barbara Sleep Disorders Medical Center
Pueblo at Bath
PO Box 689
Santa Barbara, CA 93102

Sleep Disorders Clinic
Stanford University
401 Quarry Road
Stanford, CA 94305

Southern California Sleep Apnea Center*
Lombard Medical Group
2230 Lynn Road
Thousand Oaks, CA 91360

Torrance Memorial Medical Center
Sleep Disorders Center
3330 West Lomita Boulevard
Torrance, CA 90505

Sleep Disorders Laboratory*
Kaweah Delta District Hospital
400 West Mineral King Avenue
Visalia, CA 93291

West Hills Sleep Disorders Center
23101 Sherman Place, Suite 108
West Hills, CA 91307

National Jewish/University of Colorado
Sleep Center
1400 Jackson Street, A200
Denver, CO 80206

Sleep Disorders Center
Presbyterian/St. Luke's Medical Center
1719 East 19th Avenue
Denver, CO 80218

New Haven Sleep Disorders Center
100 York Street
University Towers
New Haven, CT 06511

Sibley Memorial Hospital Sleep Disorders Center
5255 Loughboro Road Northwest
Washington, DC 20016

Sleep Disorders Center
Georgetown University Hospital
3800 Reservoir Road, NW
Washington, DC 20007-2197

Boca Raton Sleep Disorders Center
899 Meadows Road, Suite 101
Boca Raton, FL 33486

Sleep Disorder Laboratory*
Broward General Medical Center
1600 South Andrews Avenue
Fort Lauderdale, FL 33316

Sleep Disorders Center
Baptist Medical Center
The Nemours Children's Clinic
800 Prudential Drive
Jacksonville, FL 32207

Center for Sleep Disordered Breathing*
PO Box 2982
Jacksonville, FL 32203

Mayo Sleep Disorders Center
Mayo Clinic Jacksonville
4500 San Pablo Road
Jacksonville, FL 32224

Watson Clinic Sleep Disorders Center
The Watson Clinic
1600 Lakeland HIlls Boulevard, PO Box 95000
Lakeland, FL 33804-5000

Atlantic Sleep Disorders Center
1401 South Apollo Boulevard
Melbourne, FL 32901

Sleep Disorders Center
Mt. Sinai medical Center
4300 Alton Road
Miami Beach, FL 33140

Sleep Disorders Center
Miami Children's Hospital
6125 Southwest 31st Street
Miami, FL 33155

The University of Miami School of Medicine, JMMC
and VA Medical Center Sleep Disorders Center
The University of Miami
1201 Northwest 16th Street, Suite A240 (D4-5)
Miami, FL 33125

Florida Hospital Sleep Disorders Center
601 East Rollins Avenue
Orlando, FL 32803

Sleep Disorders Center
Sarasota Memorial Hospital
1700 South Tamiami Trail
Sarasota, FL 34239

St. Petersburg Sleep Disorders Center
2525 Pasadena Avenue South, Suite S
St. Petersburg, FL 33707

Atlanta Center for Sleep Disorders
Georgia Baptist Medical Center
303 Parkway, PO Box 44
Atlanta, GA 30312

Sleep Disorders Center
Northside Hospital
1000 Johnson Ferry Road
Atlanta, GA 30342

Sleep Disorders Center of Georgia
5505 Peachtree Dunwoody Road, Suite 370
Atlanta, GA 30342

Department of Sleep Disorders Medicine
Candler Hospital
5353 Reynolds Street
Savannah, GA 31405

Sleep Disorders Center
Memorial Medical Center, Inc.
4700 Waters Avenue
Savannah, GA 31403

Savannah Sleep Disorders Center
Saint Joseph's Hospital
#6 St. Joseph's Professional Plaza
11706 Mercy Boulevard
Savannah, GA 31419

Pulmonary Sleep Disorders Center*
Kuakini Medical Center
347 North Kuakini Street
Honolulu, HI 96817

Sleep Disorders Center of the Pacific
Straub Clinic & Hospital
888 South King Street
Honolulu, HI 96813

Sleep Disorders Center
Genesis Medical Center
1401 West Central park
Davenport, IA 52804

Sleep Disorders Center
The Department of Neurology
The University of Iowa Hospitals and Clinics
Iowa City, IA 52242

Sleep Disorder Service and Research Center
Rush-Presbyterian-St. Luke's
1653 West Congress Parkway
Chicago, IL 60612

Sleep Disorders Center
The University of Chicago Hospitals
5841 South Maryland
MC2091
Chicago, IL 60637

Sleep Disorders Center
Evanston Hospital
2650 Ridge Avenue
Evanston, IL 60201

C. Duane Morgan Sleep Disorders Center
Methodist Medical Center of Illinois
221 Northeast Glen Oak Avenue
Peoria, IL 61636

SIU School of Medicine/Memorial Medical Center
Sleep Disorders Center
80 North Rutledge
Springfield, IL 62781

Carle Regional Sleep Disorders Center
611 West Park Street
Urbana, IL 61801-2595

St. Mary's Sleep Disorders Center*
St. Mary's Medical Center
3700 Washington Avenue
Evansville, IN 47750

St. Joseph Sleep Disorders Center
St. Joseph Medical Center
700 Broadway
Fort Wayne, IN 46802

Sleep/Wake Disorders Center
Community Hospitals of Indianapolis
1500 North Ritter Avenue
Indianapolis, IN 46219

Sleep Disorders Center
Winona Memorial Hospital
3232 North Meridian Street
Indianapolis, IN 46208

Sleep Alertness Center
Lafayette Home Hospital
2400 South Street
Lafayette, IN 47904

Sleep Disorders Center
Good Samaritan Hospital
520 South 7th Street
Vincennes, IN 47591

Sleep Disorders Center
St. Francis Hospital and Medical Center
1700 Southwest 7th Street
Topeka, KS 66606-1690

Sleep Disorders Center
Wesley Medical Center
550 North Hillside
Wichita, KS 67214-4976

Sleep Lab*
The Medical Center at Bowling Green
250 Park Street
PO Box 90010
Bowling Green, KY 42101-9010

Appendix A

The Sleep Disorder Center of St. Luke Hospital
St. Luke Hospital, Inc.
85 North Grand Avenue
Fort Thomas, KY 41075

Sleep Apnea Center
Good Samaritan Hospital
310 South Limestone
Lexington, KY 40508

Sleep Disorders Center
St. Joseph's Hospital
One St. Joseph Drive
Lexington, KY 40504

Sleep Disorders Center
Audubon Regional Medical Center
One Audubon Plaza Drive
Louisville, KY 40217

Mercy + Baptist Sleep Disorders Center
Mercy + Baptist Medical Center
2700 Napoleon Avenue
New Orleans, LA 70115

Tulane Sleep Disorders Center
1415 Tulane Avenue
New Orleans, LA 70112

LSU Sleep Disorders Center
Louisiana State University Medical Center
PO Box 33932
Shreveport, LA 71130-3932

Sleep Disorders Center
Beth Israel Hospital
330 Brookline Avenue KS430
Boston, MA 02215

Sleep Disorders Center
Lahey Clinic
41 Mall Road
Burlington, MA 01805

Maryland Sleep Disorders Center, Inc.
Ruxton Towers, Suite 211
8415 Bellona Lane
Baltimore, MD 21204

The Johns Hopkins Sleep Disorders Center
Asthma and Allergy Building, Room 4B50
Johns Hopkins Bayview Medical Center
Johns Hopkins Bayview Circle
Baltimore, MD 21224

Shady Grove Sleep Disorders Center
14915 Broschart Road
Suite 102
Rockville, MD 20850

Sleep Laboratory*
Maine Medical Center
22 Bramhall Street
Portland, ME 04102

Sleep/Wake Disorders Unit (127B)
VA Medical Center
Southfield & Outer Drive
Allen Park, MI 48101

Sleep Disorders Center
University of Michigan Hospitals
1500 East Medical Center Drive
Med Inn c433
Box 0842
Ann Arbor, MI 48109-0115

Sleep Disorders Center
Catherine McAuley Health Systems
PO Box 995
Ann Arbor, MI 48106

Sleep Disorders Clinic
Bay Medical Center
1900 Columbus Avenue
Bay City, MI 48708

Sleep Disorders Center
Henry Ford Hospital
2799 West Grand Boulevard
Detroit, MI 48202

Sleep Disorders Center
Butterworth Hospital
100 Michigan Street Northeast
Grand Rapids, MI 49503

Sleep Disorders Center
Michigan Capital Medical Center-Pennsylvania Campus
2727 South Pennsylvania Avenue
Lansing, MI 48910

Michigan Capital Healthcare
Sleep/Wake Center
2025 South Washington Avenue
Suite 300
Lansing, MI 48910-0817

Sleep Disorders Center
Oakwood Downriver Medical Center
25750 West Outer Drive
Lincoln Park, MI 48146-1599

Sleep & Respiratory Associates of Michigan
28200 Franklin Road
Southfield, MI 48034

Munson Sleep Disorders Center
Munson Medical Center
1105 6th Street
MPB Suite 307
Traverse City, MI 49684-2386

Sleep Disorders Institute
44199 Dequindre, Suite 311
Troy, MI 48098

Duluth Regional Sleep Disorders Center
St. Mary's Medical Center
407 East Third Street
Duluth, MN 55805

Sleep Disorders Center
Abbott Northwestern Hospital
800 East 28th Street at Chicago Avenue
Minneapolis, MN 55407

Minnesota Regional Sleep Disorders Center, #867B
Hennepin County Medical Center
701 Park Avenue South
Minneapolis, MN 55415

Mayo Sleep Disorders Center
Mayo Clinic
200 First Street Southwest
Rochester, MN 55905

Sleep Disorders Center
Methodist Hospital
6500 Excelsior Boulevard
St. Louis Park, MN 55426

University of Missouri Sleep Disorders Center
M-741 Neurology
University Hospital and Clinics
One Hospital Drive
Columbia, MO 65212

Sleep Disorders Center
Research Medical Center
2316 East Meyer Boulevard
Kansas City, MO 64132-1199

Sleep Disorders Center
St. Luke's Hospital
4400 Wornall Road
Kansas City, MO 64111

Cox Regional Sleep Disorders Center
3800 South National Avenue
Suite LL 150
Springfield, MO 65807

Sleep Disorders Center
St. Louis University Medical Center
1221 South Grand Boulevard
St. Louis, MO 63104

Sleep Disorders & Research Center
Deaconess Medical Center
6150 Oakland Avenue
St. Louis, MO 63139

Sleep Disorders Center
Memorial Hospital at Gulfport
PO Box 1810
Gulfport, MS 39501

Appendix A

Sleep Disorders Center
Forrest General Hospital
PO Box 16389
6051 Highway 49
Hattiesburg, MS 39404

Sleep Disorders Center
University of MIssissippi Medical Center
2500 North State Street
Jackson, MS 39216-4505

Sleep Medicine Center of Asheville
1091 Hendersonville Road
Asheville, NC 28803

Sleep Center
University Hospital
PO Box 560727, 8800 North Tyron Street
Charlotte, NC 28256

Sleep Disorders Center
The Moses H. Cone Memorial Hospital
1200 North Elm Street
Greensboro, NC 27401-1020

Summit Sleep Disorders Center
160 Charlois Boulevard
Winston-Salem, NC 27103

Sleep Disorders Center
MeritCare Hospital
720 4th Street North
Fargo, ND 58122

Great Plains Regional Sleep Physiology Center
Lincoln General Hospital
2300 South 16th Street
Lincoln, NE 68502

Sleep Disorders Center
Methodist/Richard Young Hospital
2566 St. Mary's Avenue
Omaha, NE 68105

Sleep Disorders Center
Bishop Clarkson Memorial Hospital
44th and Dewey
Omaha, NE 68105-1018

Sleep-Wake Disorders Center
Hampstead Hospital
East Road
Hampstead, NH 03841

Sleep Disorders Center
Dartmouth-Hitchcock Medical Center
One Medical Center Drive
Lebanon, NH 03756

Comprehensive Sleep Disorders Center
Robert Wood Johnson University Hospital/
UMDNJ - Robert Wood Johnson Medical School
One Robert Wood Johnson Place, PO Box 2601
New Brunswick, NJ 08903-2601

Appendix A

Sleep Disorders Center
Newark Beth Israel Medical Center
201 Lyons Avenue
Newark, NJ 07112

Mercer Medical Center Sleep Disorders Center
Mercer Medical Center
446 Bellevue Avenue
PO Box 1658
Trenton, NJ 08607

University Hospital Sleep Disorders Center
University of New Mexico Hospital
4775 Indian School Road Northeast
Suite 307
Albuquerque, NM 87110

Regional Center for Sleep Disorders
Sunrise Hospital and Medical Center
3186 South Maryland Parkway
Las Vegas, NV 89109

Washoe Sleep Disorders Center and Laboratory
Washoe Professional Building and Medical Center
75 Pringle Way
Suites 701-702
Reno, NV 89502

Capital Region Sleep/Wake Disorders Center
St. Peter's Hospital and Albany Medical Center
25 Hackett Boulevard
Albany, NY 12208

Sleep-Wake Disorders Center
Montefiore Medical Center
111 East 210th Street
Bronx, NY 10467

Sleep Disorders Center
Winthrop-University Hospital
222 Station Plaza North
Mineola, NY 11501

Sleep-Wake Disorders Center
Long Island Jewish Medical Center
270-05 76th Avenue
New Hyde Park, NY 11042

The Sleep Disorders Center
Columbia Presbyterian Medical Center
161 Fort Washington Avenue
New York, NY 10032

Sleep Disorders Institute
St. Luke's/Roosevelt Hospital Center
Amsterdam Avenue at 114th Street
New York, NY 10025

Sleep Disorders Center of Rochester
2110 Clinton Avenue South
Rochester, NY 14618

Sleep Disorders Center
State University of New York at Stony Brook
University Hospital, MR 120 A
Stony Brook, NY 11794-7139

The Sleep Laboratory*
St. Joseph's Hospital Health Center
301 Prospect Avenue
Syracuse, NY 13203

The Sleep Center
Community General Hospital
Broad Road
Syracuse, NY 13215

Sleep-Wake Disorders Center
New York Hospital-Cornell Medical Center
21 Bloomingdale Road
White Plains, NY 10605

The Center for Research in Sleep Disorders
Affiliated with Mercy Hospital of Hamilton/Fairfield
1275 East Kemper Road
Cincinnati, OH 45246

Sleep Disorders Center
Bethesda Oak Hospital
619 Oak Street
Cincinnati, OH 45206

Sleep Disorders Center
The Cleveland Clinic Foundation
9500 Euclid Avenue
Desk S-83
Cleveland, OH 44195

Sleep Disorders Center
Case Western Reserve University
2101 Adelbert Road
Cleveland, OH 44106

Sleep Disorders Center
The Ohio State University Hospitals
Rhodes Hall, S1032
410 West 10th Avenue
Columbus, OH 43210-1228

The Center for Sleep & Wake Disorders
Miami Valley Hospital
One Wyoming Street
Suite G-200
Dayton, OH 45409

Ohio Sleep Medicine Institute
4975 Bradenton Avenue
Dublin, OH 43017

Sleep Disorders Center
Kettering Medical Center
3535 Southern Boulevard
Kettering, OH 45429-1295

Sleep Disorders Center
St. Vincent Medical Center
2213 Cherry Street
Toledo, OH 43608-2691

Northwest Ohio Sleep Disorders Center
The Toledo Hospital
Harris-McIntosh Tower, Second Floor
2142 North Cove Boulevard
Toledo, OH 43606

Sleep Disorders Center
Good Samaritan Medical Center
800 Forest Avenue
Zanesville, OH 43701

Sleep Disorders Center
Sacred Heart General Hospital
1255 Hilyard Street
PO Box 10905
Eugene, OR 97440

Sleep Disorders Center
Rogue Valley Medical Center
2825 East Barnett Road
Medford, OR 97504

Sleep Disorders Laboratory*
Providence Medical Center
4805 Northeast Glisan Street
Portland, OR 97213

Pacific Northwest Sleep Disorders Program
1849 Northwest Kearney Street
Suite 202
Portland, OR 97210

Salem Hospital Sleep Disorders Center
Salem Hospital
665 Winter Street Southeast
Salem, OR 97309-5014

Sleep Disorders Center
Lower Bucks Hospital
501 Bath Road
Bristol, PA 19007

Sleep Disorders Center*
The Good Samaritan Medical Center
1020 Franklin Street
Johnstown, PA 15905

Sleep Disorders Center of Lancaster
Lancaster General Hospital
555 North Duke Street
Lancaster, PA 17604-3555

Penn Center for Sleep Disorders
Hospital of the University of Pennsylvania
3400 Spruce Street, 11 Gates West
Philadelphia, PA 19104

Sleep Disorders Center
Thomas Jefferson University
1025 Walnut Street
Suite 316
Philadelphia, PA 19107

Appendix A

Sleep Disorders Center
The Medical College of Pennsylvania
3200 Henry Avenue
Philadelphia, PA 19129

Sleep and Chronobiology Center
Western Psychiatric Institute and Clinic
3811 O'Hara Street
Pittsburgh, PA 15213-2593

Pulmonary Sleep Evaluation Center*
Montefiore University Hospital
3459 Fifth Avenue, S639
Pittsburgh, PA 15213

Sleep Disorders Center
Community Medical Center
1822 Mulberry Street
Scranton, PA 18510

Sleep Disorders Center
Crozer-Chester Medical Center
One Medical Center Boulevard
Upland, PA 19013-3975

Sleep Disorders Center
The Lankenau Hospital
100 Lancaster Avenue
Wynnewood, PA 19096

Sleep Disorders Center
Rhode Island Hospital
593 Eddy Street, APC-301
Providence, RI 02903

Roper Sleep/Wake Disorders Center
Roper Hospital
316 Calhoun Street
Charleston, SC 29401-1125

Sleep Disorders Center of South Carolina
Baptist Medical Center
Taylor at Marion Streets
Columbia, SC 29220

Sleep Disorders Center of the Greenville Hospital System
Greenville Memorial Hospital
701 Grove Road
Greenville, SC 29605

Children's Sleep Disorders Center*
Self Memorial Hospital
1325 Spring Street
Greenwood, SC 29646

Sleep Disorders Center
Spartanburg Regional Medical Center
101 East Wood Street
Spartanburg, SC 29303

Appendix A

The Sleep Center
Rapid City Regional Hospital
353 Fairmont Boulevard
PO Box 6000
Rapid City, SD 57709

Sleep Disorders Center
Sioux Valley Hospital
1100 South Euclid
Sioux Falls, SD 57117-5039

Sleep Disorders Laboratory*
HCA Regional Hospital of Jackson
367 Hospital Boulevard
Jackson, TN 38303

Sleep Disorders Center
Ft. Sanders Regional Medical Center
1901 West Clinch Avenue
Knoxville, TN 37916

Sleep Disorders Center
St. Mary's Medical Center
900 East Oak Hill Avenue
Knoxville, TN 37917-4556

BMH Sleep Disorders Center
Baptist Memorial Hospital
899 Madison Avenue
Memphis, TN 38146

Methodist Sleep Disorders Center
Methodist Hospital of Memphis
1265 Union Avenue (12 Thomas)
Memphis, TN 38104

Sleep Disorders Center
Saint Thomas Hospital
PO Box 380
Nashville, TN 37202

Sleep Disorders Center
Centennial Medical Center
2300 Patterson Street
Nashville, TN 37203

NWTH Sleep Disorders Center
Northwest Texas Hospital
PO Box 1110
Amarillo, TX 79175

Sleep Medicine Institute
Presbyterian Hospital of Dallas
8200 Walnut Hill Lane
Dallas, TX 75231

Sleep Disorders Center for Children
Children's Medical Center of Dallas
1935 Motor Street
Dallas, TX 75235

Appendix A

Sleep Disorders Center
Providence Memorial Hospital
2001 North Oregon
El Paso, TX 79902

Sleep Disorders Center
Columbia Medical Center West
1801 North Oregon
El Paso, TX 79902

All Saints Sleep Disorders Diagnostic & Treatment Center
All Saints Episcopal Hospital
1400 8th Avenue
Fort Worth, TX 76104

Center for Sleep Related Breathing Disorders*
Hermann Hospital
6411 Fannin
Houston, TX 77030

Sleep Disorders Center
Spring Branch Medical Center
8850 Long Point Road
Suite 420 S
Houston, TX 77055

Sleep Disorders Center
Department of Psychiatry
Baylor College of Medicine and VA Medical Center
One Baylor Plaza
Houston, TX 77030

Sleep Disorders Center
Scott and White Clinic
2401 South 31st Street
Temple, TX 76508

University of Utah Hospital Sleep Disorders Center
University of Utah Hospital
50 North Medical Drive
Salt Lake City, UT 84132

Intermountain Sleep Disorders Center
LDS Hospital
325 8th Avenue
Salt Lake City, UT 84143

Sleep Disorders Center
Eastern Virginia Medical School
Sentara Norfolk General Hospital
600 Gresham Drive
Norfolk, VA 23507

Sleep Disorders Center
Chippenham Medical Center
7101 Jahnke Road
Richmond, VA 23225

Sleep Disorders Center
Medical College of Virginia
PO Box 710 - MCV
Richmond, VA 23298-0710

Sleep Disorders Center
Community Hospital of Roanoke Valley
PO Box 12946
Roanoke, VA 24029

Sleep Disorders Center for Southwest Washington
St. Peter Hospital
413 North Lilly Road
Olympia, WA 98506

Richland Sleep Laboratory*
800 Swift Boulevard
Suite 220
Richland, WA 99352

Providence Sleep Disorders Center
Jefferson Tower
Suite 203
1600 East Jefferson
Seattle, WA 98122

Seattle Sleep Disorders Center
Swedish Medical Center/Ballard
NW Market and Barnes
Seattle, WA 98107-1507

Sleep Disorders Center
Sacred Heart Doctors Building
105 West Eighth Avenue
Suite 418
Spokane, WA 99204

St. Clare Sleep Related Breathing Disorders Clinic*
St. Clare Hospital
11315 Bridgeport Way Southwest
Tacoma, WA 98499

Regional Sleep Disorders Center
Appleton Medical Center
1818 North Meade Street
Appleton, WI 54911

St. Vincent Hospital Sleep Disorders Center
St. Vincent Hospital
PO Box 13508
Green Bay, WI 54307-3508

Wisconsin Sleep Disorders Center
Gundersen Clinic, Ltd.
1836 South Avenue
La Crosse, WI 54601

Comprehensive Sleep Disorders Center
B6/579 Clinical Science Center
University of Wisconsin Hospitals and Clinics
600 Highland Avenue
Madison, WI 53792

Sleep Disorders Center
Marshfield Clinic
1000 North Oak Avenue
Marshfield, WI 54449

St. Luke's Sleep Disorders Center
St. Luke's Medical Center
2900 West Oklahoma Avenue
Milwaukee, WI 53201-2901

Sleep/Wake Disorders Center
St. Mary's Hospital
2320 North Lake Drive
PO Box 503
Milwaukee, WI 53201-4565

Milwaukee Regional Sleep Disorders Center
Columbia Hospital
2025 East Newport Avenue
Milwaukee, Wi 53211

Sleep Disorders Center
Charleston Area Medical Center
501 Morris Street - PO Box 1393
Charleston, WV 25325

Appendix B

The L-tryptophan Disaster

Z Z Z Z Z Z Z Z Z Z Z Z Z Z Z Z Z Z Z Z Z Z Z

After spending most of my life in what I now realize was a sleep-deprived state, I began taking L-tryptophan to enhance my levels of the brain chemical serotonin. The results were so remarkable that I began treating other women who were suffering the devastating symptoms of this syndrome. My own experience with this amino acid prompted me to write my first book, *The Pre-Menstrual Solution.*

In 1989, several years after I published my book, disaster struck. Showa Denko, a Japanese manufacturer of this amino acid, streamlined the processing techniques in making L-tryptophan. According to the Center for Disease Control, this switch caused a contamination in <u>specific</u> batches of the amino acid that resulted in a score of fatalities and at least a thousand cases of what has since been known as Eosinophilia Myalgia Syndrome (EMS). Shortly thereafter, the FDA instituted a peremptory ban on L-tryptophan, and overnight, this immensely useful natural sleep enhancer disappeared from the shelves of health food stores all over the country.

As terrible as the tragedy of EMS may have been, I believe that L-tryptophan does not deserve this fate. This amino acid had been on the domestic market for over 20 years, and there are thousands of studies, published in respected medical journals, to support its safety and effectiveness. But no one in the United States can buy it today.

In Canada, on the other hand, as well as many other countries overseas, L-tryptophan is still legally available. In Canada, it is available by prescription under the name Tryptan. ICN Canada, which is the sole Canadian distributor, did not buy its supplies from Showa Denko. It is hardly a coincidence that Canadian authorities have not reported a single case of EMS inside their borders. Instead of pulling this valuable drug from the market, Canada is currently conducting studies to expand its therapeutic applications. And I know for a fact that thousands of consumers I have been in contact with over the years are now obtaining their supply of L-tryptophan from Canada. Unfortunately, the cost of this product to America is very high. WARNING: DO NOT TAKE L-TRYPTOPHAN

FROM THE UNITED STATES AS IT MAY STILL BE CONTAMINATED.

I feel betrayed by my own government in this regard, as do, I am sure, many other Americans. I WOULD URGE THE FOOD AND DRUG ADMINISTRATION TO ADOPT POLICIES THAT WOULD PREVENT THIS KIND OF CONTAMINATION FROM HAPPENING AGAIN, WHILE ALLOWING CITIZENS AND THE MEDICAL COMMUNITY THE FREEDOM TO CONTINUE TO USE THIS VITAL NUTRIENT. I believe that it is the responsibility of the FDA to adopt guidelines that would prevent this kind of fiasco from happening again. There are thousands of people who believe that the quality of their lives has been severely effected by the current FDA policy which does not allow the sale of pure L-tryptophan.

I urge each and every one of you who wish to be able to obtain L-tryptophan in your own country to personally call your senator and congressman and demand that this matter be investigated. You can also write letters to your favorite talk shows demanding that this topic be discussed. We have the power to change this situation. The power to enjoy a good night's sleep. Let's use it!

Appendix B

Send a letter to the FDA with a cc to the White House:

Food & Drug Administration
Attn: David Kessler
5600 Fishers Lane
Rockville, MD 20857
(301) 443-3170

Call the following numbers to get your congressional representative's name and address:

House & Senate - (202) 225-3121

Call the network to get the address of your favorite talk show:

ABC
77 W. 66th Street
New York, NY 10023
(212) 456-7777

CBS
524 W. 57th Street
New York, NY 10019
(212) 975-4321

NBC
31 Rockefeller Plaza
New York, NY 10112
(212) 664-4444

Appendix C

The Biochemistry of Sleep

Z Z Z Z Z Z Z Z Z Z Z Z Z Z Z Z Z Z Z Z Z Z Z Z Z

I, and other researchers, believe that serotonin is the key to mental well being and, perhaps, even criminal behavior, drug and alcohol addiction and mental illness. I certainly believe it is the cause of premenstrual syndrome in women.

What Is Serotonin?

Serotonin is a chemical that is present in both your brain and your body's circulating system. This holds true for men, women, and children. It must be noted, however, that the circulating serotonin does not pass into the brain, nor does the brain serotonin pass into the circulating system. There are two separate systems of serotonin, and, thus, they are not interchangeable.

Brain serotonin is a neurotransmitter or brain chemical messenger. This is important because serotonin has many functions in the brain. It regulates dietary cravings, the quality and quantity of sleep, and it is important in female hormone production. Because it's a neurotransmitter, or brain chemical messenger, it helps to transmit messages from one part of the brain to another. If a person has low levels of serotonin, messages don't get through as rapidly. This is why so many people you encounter during a normal work day may seem confused or out of sorts.

Exactly What Are Amino Acids?

There are 22 amino acids. Of the 22 amino acids, our body has the ability to make all but eight. Of course, it's essential that we have all the basic building blocks to make the other 14. But eight of them must be obtained from the diet. Without these amino acids, human life cannot survive. Hence, their presence in the diet is mandatory, and dietary protein is actually judged on its contents of those eight amino acids.

Tryptophan is among those essential amino acids that must be replaced daily in the diet, as the body does not have the ability to store it. Because L-tryptophan is necessary to make serotonin, this also means that serotonin must be replaced daily in the body. Aside from being involved in the sleep cycle, the reproductive cycle, and dietary cravings, serotonin is an important factor in depression, a variety of physical symptoms and a healthy, happy state of mind.

Some of the factors that influence the synthesis and the metabolism of serotonin are liver function and the general availability of tryptophan in the diet. Although it is, as we have discovered, a neurotransmitter, serotonin does not cross into the brain directly. L-tryptophan enters the brain by attaching itself to a carrier molecule, much like a hitch hiker catching a ride into the brain.

Because of serotonin's strong link to emotional and social behavior, it has a significant bearing in the treatment of depression. Many anti-depressant medications are effective because they significantly increase brain serotonin levels.

Prozac is an example of an anti-depressant that selectively increases brain serotonin. Prozac accomplishes this by making serotonin available for a longer period of time in the brain. L-tryptophan, on the other hand, accomplishes an increase in brain serotonin levels by making more of the raw materials available to make brain serotonin.

The Pineal Gland and Melatonin

The regulation of sleep takes place in a part of the brain called the pineal gland, which is an obscure organ that is very near the center of the brain. Named because of the resemblance to a pine cone, the human pineal is smaller and weighs less than an aspirin. Its existence was chronicled by the early Greek anatomists, but there have been sharp disagreements over the function ever since the 4th century B.C. Herophilus suggested that the pineal was the sphincter of thought, the mind's valve. Rene Descartes, the 17th century French philosopher, went him one better when he called the pineal the seat of the rational soul.

It is in the pineal where the hormone melatonin is manufactured. It is one of the chemicals that induces people to become sleepy and experience both REM and non-REM sleep. Although sleep research is still in it's infancy, this is what we think happens when you feel you're about to drop off for the night. During the daytime, when your eye or optic nerve is perceiving daylight, your brain stores serotonin for later use in the sleep cycle. But when your optic nerve perceives darkness, serotonin is rapidly converted into the chemical, melatonin. During the day, light inhibits melatonin production in the pineal, but the gland is not idle. From dawn to dusk, it converts the amino acid, L-tryptophan, into serotonin, the substance that will be turned into melatonin at night.

The melatonin is acted upon nightly by other chemicals and enzymes. In a two-step process, serotonin is changed into melatonin and released into the bloodstream which causes drowsiness, then sleep. This entire process is activated by the way your eyes perceive light and dark. Other chemicals that are also necessary in the production of a normal night's sleep include acetylcholine and norepinepherine, to name a few. Certain vitamins, minerals and amino acids are necessary in order to enhance these chemicals.

When you awaken in the morning and your eyes perceive light, melatonin is rapidly converted back into serotonin. This causes me to wonder about the inevitable changes that must have taken place since the time when our ancestors went to sleep when the sun went down and rose when the sun came up. This was long before electricity gave us the kind of control over our sleeping habits we enjoy today.

How Serotonin Relates to PMS and Other
Symptoms of Sleep Deprivation.

For women with premenstrual syndrome, the
following symptoms appear to be a problem:
fatigue, restless sleep, insomnia, forgetfulness,
mood swings, aggression, rage, paranoia, confusion, despair, crying, decreased energy, panic,
irritability, depression, difficulty coping,
increased sexual drive, possibility of increased
episodes of herpes simplex, seizures, asthma and
migraine headaches. As you can see, many of
these symptoms are not limited to women with
premenstrual syndrome, and many people who
suffer from sleep deprivation will also experience many of the above mentioned symptoms.

These symptoms relate to serotonin for the following reasons. As the neurotransmitter serotonin is linked to behavior and mood changes, it is
also necessary for conversion to melatonin and
normal sleep. Lack of Stage 5, REM sleep can
also cause these symptoms. For example,
patients with a history of asthma, migraines or
seizures are more apt to have episodes of these
illnesses after they have been sleep deprived. In
its role as a neurotransmitter, serotonin helps
transmit messages from one part of the brain to
the other. Low levels of brain serotonin may

cause a delay in the messages getting through rapidly, causing a feeling of mental confusion and a lack of general mental clarity.

Other symptoms which women with PMS have also described are what I call physical symptoms. These symptoms would include things like bloating, breast tenderness, water retention, etc. Because serotonin is critical in terms of the timing of ovulation, low levels may cause early ovulation and a shift in estrogen/progesterone patterns. This shift in the normal estrogen/progesterone patterns can cause the above mentioned symptoms.

Other symptoms which have been related to PMS and other illnesses would include bruising easily. Since we know that serotonin promotes platelet aggregation and is important in the clotting mechanism, this means it could prevent this symptom. Those with low levels of serotonin may find that they bruise more easily. (For more information on PMS see *THE PRE-MEN-STRUAL SOLUTION, How to Tame the Shrew in You* by Jo Ann Friedrich—order form in back of book.)

Serotonin is also a factor in the treatment of migraine headaches, because sleep deprivation can intensify these headaches. But with migraine headaches, there is also vasodilation which means that the vessels are dilating. Since serotonin is also a powerful vasoconstrictor, it can help abolish these symptoms. It has been my experience that migraine headaches can be completely eliminated through a program of sleep hygiene and serotonin enhancement.

I believe that the impact of serotonin is yet to be fully recognized. Prior to its ban, the food supplement L-tryptophan was being recommended as a treatment for sufferers of migraine headaches, chronic headaches, lower back pain and arthritis. In addition, it had also been used effectively to treat childhood bedwetting, depression, drug withdrawal and a multitude of other ailments.

Serotonin and Carbohydrate Cravings

When my own PMS was severe, and I was extremely sleep deprived, food was the solace I often turned to. I found that my cravings for sugar and chocolate, as well as other carbohydrates, were so severe, that it did not matter to me, at all, that I was consuming too large a quantity of sugar. I simply had to have it. Why? Because the craving for carbohydrates or protein is directly related to the levels of serotonin in the brain. Serotonin actually controls whether we crave carbohydrates or protein. If the levels of neuroserotonin are too low, the brain tells the body to eat carbohydrates to raise these levels. As I mentioned earlier in this text, tryptophan is necessary in order to make serotonin. It would then seem logical that if we wanted to increase the amount of brain serotonin, it would be necessary to consume more protein which is rich in tryptophan and other amino acids. However, this is not the case. (For more visual clarification, please refer to Diagram 3, Chapter 8.)

Here is how the brain controls our dietary cravings. When a person ingests a protein which contains all the essential amino acids, including tryptophan, these amino acids then move from the stomach into the intestine and are absorbed into the bloodstream. These amino acids now have to compete with each other to cross what is known as the blood brain barrier. The blood brain barrier is actually our body's way of protecting us from absorbing things such as poisons. The blood brain barrier makes it difficult for us to move certain things from our bloodstream into our brain, thus, protecting the brain. All of the amino acids, which are now in our bloodstream, must compete with each other in order to cross this blood brain barrier. The problem here, however, is that the competition can be fierce. All the amino acids, including tryptophan, are trying to push each other to get in through the blood brain barrier.

Researchers at MIT found that when individuals were given a meal high in carbohydrates which caused a surge of insulin in the body, all of the amino acids, with the exception of tryptophan, became literally paralyzed. Tryptophan has the unique ability to attach itself to a carrier molecule that insulates it from insulin. And it is the only amino acid that can accomplish this. Imagine if there were 100 people in a room and all of them were trying to get out of the same doorway at the same time, the competition would be incredible and very few people would actually make it through that doorway. On the other hand, if 99 people were paralyzed, the one person who was not paralyzed would easily walk through the door. As a result, although there are no greater levels of tryptophan in the bloodstream, more becomes available to slide through the blood brain barrier, simply because the competition has been effectively eliminated. Thus, when you eat a carbohydrate, whether it be a simple one such as candy or a complex one such as a whole grain, the amount of tryptophan that crosses the brain is increased. Because simple carbohydrates tend to increase insulin levels more quickly, it is my belief that those who crave carbohydrates, in effect, are subconsciously trying to raise their brain serotonin levels. It was certainly my experience that eating sugar did, in fact, help my symptoms. But the improvement was very brief and transient. My body would then have to cope with the problems of my blood sugar bouncing up and down. I believe that there are many people who have chronically low levels of serotonin and who have difficulty actually normalizing these levels. They are, therefore, unable to effectively raise their level of serotonin high enough to cause them to crave protein. Supplementing with the amino acid L-tryptophan, in fact, causes an increase in brain serotonin which normalizes the dietary pattern. And thus neutralizes the cravings forever. Unfortunately, it is no longer available in the United States.

As you can see, the implications for serotonin are vast. I think the next several decades will show that this chemical is critical in all kinds of behavioral issues. Studies with mass murderers have shown that control groups have higher serotonin levels than those people who have murdered once in an impulsive way. People who have murdered once have higher levels than mass murderers who appear to have the lowest levels of the three groups. I don't believe that this is an accident. I am firmly convinced that the importance of this brain chemical will become evident over the next several decades. I can only hope that the FDA will reverse its opinion on the amino acid L-tryptophan.

Order Form

Please send me the following items:

_____ Sleep Mask - $9.95

_____ Dream Journal - $9.95

_____ Sleep/Relaxation Tapes (two tapes) - $14.95

_____ Quarterly Newsletter titled *Just ZZZZ Facts* - $24.95 per year

_____ *The Pre-menstrual Solution* Book - $14.95

_____ Sleep Matters Recipes - $9.95

_____ Information on how to book Jo Ann Cutler Friedrich, P.A. as a speaker for your next seminar or event.

_____ Information on ways you can help get L-tryptophan back in the United States market.

Please enclose $5.00 for shipping and handling. California residents include 8.25% sales tax.

To: Bright Books
       4718 Meridian Avenue, Suite 212
       San Jose, California 95118
       (408) 266-1400